A Population-Based Policy and Systems Change Approach to Prevent and Control Hypertension

Committee on Public Health Priorities to Reduce and Control Hypertension in the U.S. Population

Board on Population Health and Public Health Practice

INSTITUTE OF MEDICINE
OF THE NATIONAL ACADEMIES

THE NATIONAL ACADEMIES PRESS
Washington, D.C.
www.nap.edu

THE NATIONAL ACADEMIES PRESS   500 Fifth Street, N.W.   Washington, DC 20001

NOTICE: The project that is the subject of this report was approved by the Governing Board of the National Research Council, whose members are drawn from the councils of the National Academy of Sciences, the National Academy of Engineering, and the Institute of Medicine. The members of the committee responsible for the report were chosen for their special competences and with regard for appropriate balance.

This study was supported by Contract No. 200-2005-13434, TO 18 between the National Academy of Sciences and the Centers for Disease Control and Prevention. Any opinions, findings, conclusions, or recommendations expressed in this publication are those of the author(s) and do not necessarily reflect the view of the organizations or agencies that provided support for this project.

Library of Congress Cataloging-in-Publication Data

Institute of Medicine (U.S.). Committee on Public Health Priorities to Reduce and Control Hypertension in the U.S. Population.
  A population-based policy and systems change approach to prevent and control hypertension / Committee on Public Health Priorities to Reduce and Control Hypertension in the U.S. Population, Board on Population Health and Public Health Practice.
     p. ; cm.
  Includes bibliographical references.
  ISBN 978-0-309-14809-2 (pbk.) — ISBN 978-0-309-14810-8 (pdf) 1. Hypertension—Prevention—Government policy—United States. 2. Centers for Disease Control and Prevention (U.S.) Division for Heart Disease and Stroke Prevention. I. Title.
  [DNLM: 1. Centers for Disease Control and Prevention (U.S.) Division for Heart Disease and Stroke Prevention. 2. Hypertension—prevention & control—United States. 3. Community Health Planning—United States. 4. Health Policy—United States. 5. United States Government Agencies—United States. WG 340 N279907p 2010]
  RA645.H9N38 2010
  362.196'132—dc22
                         2010014536

Additional copies of this report are available from the National Academies Press, 500 Fifth Street, N.W., Lockbox 285, Washington, DC 20055; (800) 624-6242 or (202) 334-3313 (in the Washington metropolitan area); Internet, http://www.nap.edu.

For more information about the Institute of Medicine, visit the IOM home page at **www. iom.edu.**

The serpent has been a symbol of long life, healing, and knowledge among almost all cultures and religions since the beginning of recorded history. The serpent adopted as a logotype by the Institute of Medicine is a relief carving from ancient Greece, now held by the Staatliche Museen in Berlin.

Suggested citation: IOM (Institute of Medicine). 2010. *A Population-Based Policy and Systems Change Approach to Prevent and Control Hypertension.* Washington, DC: The National Academies Press.

*"Knowing is not enough; we must apply.
Willing is not enough; we must do."*
—Goethe

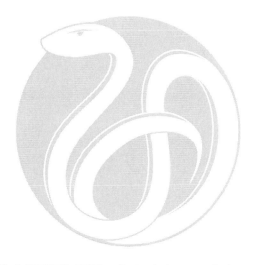

INSTITUTE OF MEDICINE
OF THE NATIONAL ACADEMIES

Advising the Nation. Improving Health.

THE NATIONAL ACADEMIES
Advisers to the Nation on Science, Engineering, and Medicine

The **National Academy of Sciences** is a private, nonprofit, self-perpetuating society of distinguished scholars engaged in scientific and engineering research, dedicated to the furtherance of science and technology and to their use for the general welfare. Upon the authority of the charter granted to it by the Congress in 1863, the Academy has a mandate that requires it to advise the federal government on scientific and technical matters. Dr. Ralph J. Cicerone is president of the National Academy of Sciences.

The **National Academy of Engineering** was established in 1964, under the charter of the National Academy of Sciences, as a parallel organization of outstanding engineers. It is autonomous in its administration and in the selection of its members, sharing with the National Academy of Sciences the responsibility for advising the federal government. The National Academy of Engineering also sponsors engineering programs aimed at meeting national needs, encourages education and research, and recognizes the superior achievements of engineers. Dr. Charles M. Vest is president of the National Academy of Engineering.

The **Institute of Medicine** was established in 1970 by the National Academy of Sciences to secure the services of eminent members of appropriate professions in the examination of policy matters pertaining to the health of the public. The Institute acts under the responsibility given to the National Academy of Sciences by its congressional charter to be an adviser to the federal government and, upon its own initiative, to identify issues of medical care, research, and education. Dr. Harvey V. Fineberg is president of the Institute of Medicine.

The **National Research Council** was organized by the National Academy of Sciences in 1916 to associate the broad community of science and technology with the Academy's purposes of furthering knowledge and advising the federal government. Functioning in accordance with general policies determined by the Academy, the Council has become the principal operating agency of both the National Academy of Sciences and the National Academy of Engineering in providing services to the government, the public, and the scientific and engineering communities. The Council is administered jointly by both Academies and the Institute of Medicine. Dr. Ralph J. Cicerone and Dr. Charles M. Vest are chair and vice chair, respectively, of the National Research Council.

www.national-academies.org

COMMITTEE ON PUBLIC HEALTH PRIORITIES TO REDUCE AND CONTROL HYPERTENSION IN THE U.S. POPULATION

DAVID W. FLEMING *(Chair, March 2009-February 2010)*, Director and Health Officer, Public Health-Seattle & King County, Seattle, WA

HOWARD KOH *(Chair, January-March 2009)*, Professor of the Practice of Public Health, Department of Health Policy and Management, Harvard School of Public Health, Boston, MA

ANA V. DIEZ ROUX, Professor of Epidemiology and Director, Center for Integrative Approaches to Health Disparities, and Associate Director, Center for Social Epidemiology and Population Health, University of Michigan School of Public Health, Ann Arbor, MI

JIANG HE, Joseph S. Copes Chair and Professor, Department of Epidemiology, Tulane University, New Orleans, LA

KATHY HEBERT, Associate Professor of Medicine, Division of Cardiology and Director, Disease Management and Outcomes Research, Miller School of Medicine, University of Miami, Miami, FL

CORINNE HUSTEN, Executive Vice President for Program and Policy, Partnership for Prevention (January-October 2009) and Senior Medical Advisor, Center for Tobacco Products, Food and Drug Administration (October 2009-February 2010), Washington DC

SHERMAN A. JAMES, Susan B. King Professor of Public Policy Studies, Professor of Family and Community Medicine, Sociology and African and African-American Studies, Duke University, Durham, NC

THOMAS G. PICKERING *(deceased)*, Director of the Behavior Cardiovascular Health and Hypertension Program, Department of Medicine, Columbia University College of Physicians and Surgeons, New York, NY

GEOFFRY ROSENTHAL, Department of Pediatrics, Cardiology Division, University of Maryland Medical Center, Baltimore, MD

WALTER C. WILLETT, Fredrick John Stare Professor of Epidemiology and Nutrition, Chair, Department of Nutrition, Harvard School of Public Health, Boston, MA

IOM Staff

ROSE MARIE MARTINEZ, Director, Board on Population Health and Public Health Practice

RITA DENG, Associate Program Officer

NORA HENNESSY, Associate Program Officer

RAINA SHARMA, Senior Program Assistant

FLORENCE POILLON, Senior Editor

Reviewers

This report has been reviewed in draft form by persons chosen for their diverse perspectives and technical expertise in accordance with procedures approved by the National Research Council's Report Review Committee. The purpose of this independent review is to provide candid and critical comments that will assist the institution in making its published report as sound as possible and to ensure that the report meets institutional standards of objectivity, evidence, and responsiveness to the study charge. The review comments and draft manuscript remain confidential to protect the integrity of the deliberative process. We thank the following for their review of the report:

Lawrence J. Appel, Johns Hopkins Bloomberg School of Public Health
Valentin Fuster, Mount Sinai School of Medicine
Maxine Hayes, State of Washington, Department of Health
Christine Johnson, New York City Department of Health and Mental Hygiene
Michael Klag, Johns Hopkins Bloomberg School of Public Health
M.A. "Tonette" Krousel-Wood, Tulane University
Claude Lenfant, National Heart, Lung, and Blood Institute

Although the reviewers listed above have provided many constructive comments and suggestions, they were not asked to endorse the conclusions or recommendations, nor did they see the final draft of the report before its release. The review of the report was overseen by **Kristine M. Gebbie,**

City University of New York. Appointed by the National Research Council and the Institute of Medicine, she was responsible for making certain that an independent examination of the report was carried out in accordance with institutional procedures and that all review comments were carefully considered. Responsibility for the final content of the report rests with the author committee and the institution.

Acknowledgments

The committee acknowledges the valuable contributions made by the many persons who shared their experience and knowledge with the committee. First the committee wishes to thank **Howard Koh,** who chaired the committee before assuming responsibility as Assistant Secretary for Health. The committee appreciates the time and insight of the presenters during the public sessions: **Kathryn Gallagher, Yuling Hong, Darwin Labarthe,** and **Michael Schooley,** Centers for Disease Control and Prevention; **Aram Chobanian,** Boston University; **Eduardo Ortiz,** National Heart, Lung, and Blood Institute; **Ed Rocella,** retired National Heart, Lung, and Blood Institute; **Sonia Angell,** New York City Department of Health and Mental Hygiene; **Susan Cooper,** Tennessee Department of Health; **Barry Davis,** University of Texas School of Public Health; **Richard Cooper,** Loyola University; **Russell Luepker,** University of Minnesota; **Stephen Lim,** University of Washington; **David Goff,** Wake Forest University; and **Frank Sacks,** Harvard University. The committee also thanks **John Forman,** Brigham and Women's Hospital, for the background paper on modifiable risk factors and population attributable fractions that informed the committee's deliberations.

This report would not have been possible without the diligent assistance of technical monitors **Diane Dunet** and **Rashon Lane,** and statistician **Cathleen Gillespie,** Centers for Disease Control and Prevention. The committee thanks the staff members of the Institute of Medicine, the National Research Council, and the National Academies Press who contributed to the development, production, and dissemination of this report. The committee thanks **Rose Marie Martinez,** study director, **Rita Deng,** associate program officer, and **Nora Hennessy,** associate program officer, for their work in navigating this complex topic with the committee, **Raina Sharma** for her diligent management of the committee logistics, and **Hope Hare** for her attention to report production.

This report was made possible by the support of the Division for Heart Disease and Stroke Prevention of the Centers for Disease Control and Prevention.

Contents

TABLES AND FIGURES

Tables

Figures

Summary

In today's public health world, the term "neglected disease" conjures up obscure tropical illnesses of little relevance to contemporary practice in the United States. Yet, when one considers the actual meaning of the words, the time may be right to add hypertension to this list. Despite the magnitude of hypertension-associated morbidity and mortality and the $73 billion in annual costs to the health care system, hypertension prevention and control is only one of a number of programs competing for a total of only $54 million (2009) in the Centers for Disease Control and Prevention's (CDC's) entire Heart Disease and Stroke Prevention portfolio.

The lack of attention to hypertension goes against the objective facts. Hypertension is one of the leading causes of preventable death in the United States. In 2005, high blood pressure was responsible for about one in six deaths of U.S. adults and was the single largest risk factor for cardiovascular mortality accounting for about 45 percent of all cardiovascular deaths. Based on data from the CDC and the National Heart, Lung, and Blood Institute (NHLBI) from 1995 to 2005, the death rate from high blood pressure increased by 25 percent and the actual number of deaths rose by 56 percent (Lloyd-Jones et al., 2009).

Hypertension, defined for adults as a systolic pressure of 140 mm Hg or greater or a diastolic pressure of 90 mm Hg or higher, is highly prevalent (Chobanian et al., 2003). Approximately 73 million Americans or nearly one in three U.S. adults has hypertension (Fields et al., 2004; Lloyd-Jones et al., 2009). An additional 59 million have prehypertension, which is defined as blood pressure ranging from 120-139 mm Hg systolic and/or 80-89 mm Hg diastolic (Chobanian et al., 2003).

The risk of developing hypertension increases with age, and in older age groups it is more common than not. Based on data from the Framingham study, the lifetime risk of hypertension is estimated to be 90 percent for people with normal blood pressure at ages 55 or 65 who live to be ages 80 to 85, respectively (Cutler et al., 2007; Vasan et al., 2002).

Hypertension is costly to the health care system. It is the most common primary diagnosis in America (Chobanian et al., 2003), and it contributes to the costs of cardiovascular disease (coronary heart disease, myocardial infarction) and stroke. The American Heart Association (AHA) recently reported the direct and indirect costs of high blood pressure as a primary diagnosis as $73.4 billion for 2009 (Lloyd-Jones et al., 2009). With respect to the cost of treating hypertension, an analysis by DeVol and Bedroussian (2007) estimated that the total expenditure for the population reporting hypertension as a condition in the Medical Expenditure Panel Survey (MEPS) was $32.5 billion in 2003 (DeVol and Bedroussian, 2007). Another study estimated the total incremental annual direct expenditures for treating hypertension (the excess expenditure of treating patients with hypertension compared to patients without hypertension) to be about $55 billion in 2001 (Balu and Thomas, 2006).

Much is known about the health consequences and costs associated with hypertension (Chapters 1 and 2). Robust clinical and public health research efforts have developed safe and cost-effective nonpharmacological and pharmacological interventions (Chapters 4 and 5) to prevent, treat, and control hypertension. Nonetheless, millions of Americans continue to develop, live with, and die from hypertension because we are failing to translate our public health and clinical knowledge into effective prevention, treatment, and control programs. In the committee's view this current state is one of neglect, defined by *Merriam-Webster* as "giving insufficient attention to something that merits attention." The recommendations offered in this report outline a population-based policy and systems change approach to addressing hypertension that can be applied at the federal, state, and local level. It is time to give full attention and take concerted actions to prevent and control hypertension.

THE CHARGE TO THE COMMITTEE

The CDC Division for Heart Disease and Stroke Prevention (DHDSP) provides national leadership to reduce the burden of disease, disability, and death from heart disease and stroke. The DHDSP is co-lead, along with the NHLBI, for the Healthy People 2010 objectives related to heart disease and stroke including four objectives specific to hypertension (Table S-1).

Findings from the *Healthy People 2010 Midcourse Review* (CDC, 2006) indicated that the nation was moving away from making progress in

TABLE S-1 Healthy People 2010 Focus Area 12: Heart and Stroke, Blood Pressure Objectives

Number	Objective
12-9.	Reduce the proportion of adults with high blood pressure.
12-10.	Increase the proportion of adults with high blood pressure whose blood pressure is under control.
12-11.	Increase the proportion of adults with high blood pressure who are taking action (for example, losing weight, increasing physical activity, or reducing sodium intake) to help control their blood pressure.
12-12.	Increase the proportion of adults who have had their blood pressure measured within the preceding 2 years and can state whether their blood pressure was normal or high.

SOURCE: CDC, 2006.

the target objectives as reflected by increases in the prevalence of high blood pressure among adults and among children and adolescents. This moving away from Healthy People 2010 goals provided an increased emphasis for a DHDSP programmatic focus on hypertension.

The DHDSP has developed a strategic plan to reduce and control hypertension that recognizes the urgent need to implement known effective practices and to develop new ones. The plan identifies a number of action areas and goals for the prevention and control of hypertension. The CDC requested assistance and guidance from the Institute of Medicine (IOM) to determine a small set of high-priority areas in which public health can focus its efforts to accelerate progress in hypertension reduction and control. Specifically, the CDC requested that the IOM convene an expert committee to review available public health strategies for reducing and controlling hypertension in the U.S. population, including both science-based and practice-based knowledge. In conducting its work, the committee was asked to consider the following questions:

What are the highest-priority action areas on which CDC's Division for Heart Disease and Stroke Prevention and other partners should focus near-term efforts in hypertension?

1. Identify the particular role of CDC's DHDSP in addressing the highest-priority areas.
2. Identify the role of state health departments in advancing progress in the priority action areas.
3. Identify the role of other public health partners.

4. What visible impacts can be expected if DHDSP focuses its efforts in these priority areas?
5. What indicators should be monitored to assess the progress of DHDSP, state health departments, and partners in implementing the committee's recommendations?
6. What are the potential positive and negative impacts on health disparities that could result if the committee's recommendations are implemented?
7. What indicators should be monitored related to health disparities to ensure the intended impact of the DHDSP priority action areas identified?

The committee was not expected to conduct a new, detailed review of peer-reviewed literature on hypertension because such literature reviews, meta-analyses, and syntheses already exist and have been used to inform existing guidelines and recommendations.

FINDINGS AND RECOMMENDATIONS

The CDC, through the Division for Heart Disease and Stroke Prevention, has leveraged its broader cardiovascular disease prevention and control programmatic efforts to address hypertension primarily through its state heart disease and stoke prevention programs. Many of these efforts are described in Chapter 3 and throughout other chapters. Objectively, however, there are several significant problems with the current status and direction of hypertension prevention and control activities:

- Hypertension is only one component of a larger cardiovascular disease prevention program that, as a consequence, has more of a medical care rather than a population-based prevention focus based on system change.
- The CDC's cardiovascular disease program in general, and the hypertension program in particular, are dramatically under funded relative to the preventable burden of disease and the strategy and action plan that have been developed.

In light of the current situation, short-term programmatic priorities must be tempered by the economic reality that the absolute amount of prevention resources available to the CDC are limited, and thus cost-effectiveness and absolute costs must be considered. Compared with interventions directed toward individuals, population-based interventions and interventions directed at system improvements and efficiencies are more likely to be more practical and realistic in the current resource-constrained environment. The committee believes that the reality of limited resources for hypertension prevention requires that DHDSP shift the weight of its focus to approaches that cater to the strength of the public health system—population-based and systems approaches rather than health care-based approaches.

To that end, the committee has recommended a number of high-priority strategies to prevent and control hypertension to the CDC and DHDSP. The recommendations embody a population-based approach grounded in the principles of measurement, system change, and accountability and bridge public health and clinical care. The DHDSP can support the implementation of these recommendations in collaboration with other CDC units. In brief, the recommendations seek to:

- Shift the balance of the DHDSP hypertension priorities from individual-based strategies to population-based strategies to:
  o strengthen collaboration among CDC units (and their partners) to ensure that hypertension is included as a dimension of other population-based activities around healthy lifestyle improvement, particularly greater consumption of potassium-rich fruits and vegetables, increased physical activity, and weight management
  o strengthen CDC's leadership in monitoring and reducing sodium intake in the American diet to meet current dietary guidelines
  o improve the surveillance and reporting of hypertension to better characterize general trends and trends among subgroups of the population
- Promote policy and *system* change approaches to:
  o improve the quality of care provided to individuals by assuring that individuals who should be in treatment are in treatment and receive care that is consistent with current treatment guidelines
    ♦ increase the importance of treating systolic hypertension, especially among the elderly
  o remove economic barriers to effective antihypertensive medications
  o provide community-based support for individuals with hypertension through community health workers who are trained in dietary and physical activity counseling.

The population-based policy and systems approach recommended is not only limited to the CDC and DHDSP but also extends and applies to state and local health departments and to other partners. The high-priority recommendations directed to the DHDSP are discussed in Chapters 4 and 5 have been translated for action by state and local health jurisdictions in Chapter 6. Successfully implementing a population-based policy and systems approach at all levels will depend on the resources available and systems of accountability to ensure that resources are appropriately aligned and outcomes are achieved; those recommendations are also found in Chapter 6. For ease of presentation in this summary, the recommendations for the DHDSP and its most important partners, state and local health jurisdictions, have been integrated in this summary but are discussed separately in relevant chapters.

Population-Based Strategies

Hypertension is highly preventable and manageable through lifestyle interventions. Given the co-occurrence or association with poor diet, physical inactivity, and obesity, which appear to be on the increase, lifestyle modifications are of even greater importance. Government public health agencies are the only organizations with the mandate to provide population-wide services, and the CDC and state and local public health agencies are more experienced and skilled in population-based interventions than in interventions that provide health care directly to individuals. Through leadership and convening strategies, government public health agencies can galvanize political commitment, develop policy, prioritize funding, and coordinate programs (Baker and Porter, 2005).

A stronger focus on primary prevention of hypertension is consistent with the DHDSP's responsibility as co-lead of Healthy People 2010's focus area on heart disease and stroke and in achieving progress in reducing the proportion of adults with high blood pressure. The committee acknowledges that within the CDC, the DHDSP is not the focal point for addressing dietary imbalances, physical inactivity, and other determinants to prevent the development of risk factors and progression of high blood pressure. It also acknowledges that the focus of DHDSP activities is primarily on adults, not children. The committee is also aware that the DHDSP, through the Cardiovascular Health Collaboration of the National Center for Chronic Disease Prevention and Health Promotion, collaborates with units across the CDC. The committee believes, however, that this collaboration can be strengthened and extended to leverage the efforts and resources of those programs to ensure proper attention to the prevention of hypertension and the reduction of hypertension risk factors.

Based on the review of the literature there is strong evidence linking overweight and obesity, high sodium intake, low potassium intake, unhealthy diet, and decreased physical activity to hypertension. These risk factors contribute substantially to the burden of hypertension in the United

States; further, the prevalence of many of these risk factors is increasing. The observational and randomized clinical trial literature on interventions to reduce overweight and obesity, decrease sodium intake, support eating a healthy diet, increase potassium intake, and increase physical activity also indicate that these risk factors are modifiable and that they can help reduce blood pressure levels. The committee concludes in light of: (1) the high prevalence of these risk factors that contribute significantly to the development of high blood pressure, (2) existing interventions to reduce these risk factors, and (3) the potential to reduce the burden of hypertension if the interventions are implemented, that actions to reduce these risk factors merit a high priority. The committee recommendations follow; the number appearing before the recommendation refers to the chapter and number of the recommendation in that chapter.

4.1 The committee recommends that the Division for Heart Disease and Stroke Prevention integrate hypertension prevention and control in programmatic efforts to effect system, environmental, and policy changes through collaboration with other CDC units and their external partners, to ensure that population-based lifestyle or behavior change interventions where delivered, are delivered in a coordinated manner that includes a focus on the prevention of hypertension. High-priority programmatic activities on which to collaborate include interventions for:

- reducing overweight and obesity;
- promoting the consumption of a healthy diet that includes a higher intake of fruits, vegetables, whole grains, and unsaturated fats and reduced amounts of overall calories, sugar, sugary beverages, refined starches, and saturated and trans fats (for example, a diet that is consistent with the OmniHeart diet);
- increasing potassium-rich fruits and vegetables in the diet; and
- increasing physical activity.

4.2 The committee recommends that population-based interventions to improve physical activity and food environments (typically the focus of other CDC units) should include an evaluation of their feasibility and effectiveness, and their specific impact on hypertension prevalence and control.

4.3 To create a better balance between primary and secondary prevention of hypertension the committee recommends that the Division for Heart Disease and Stroke Prevention leverage its ability to shape state activities, through its grant making and cooperative agreements, to encourage state activities to shift toward population-based prevention of hypertension.

The committee views a population-based policy and systems approach to prevent and control hypertension at the state and local level to be consistent with the broad mandates of state and local public health jurisdictions.

6.1 The committee recommends that state and local public health jurisdictions give priority to population-wide approaches over individual-based approaches to prevent and control hypertension.

6.2 The committee recommends that state and local public health jurisdictions integrate hypertension prevention and control in programmatic efforts to effect system, environmental, and policy changes that will support healthy eating, active living, and obesity prevention. Existing and new programmatic efforts should be assessed to ensure they are aligned with populations most likely to be affected by hypertension such as older populations, which are often not the target of these programs.

Based upon 2004 statistics using calculated intakes of sodium, 87 percent of U.S. adults consumed what is considered excess sodium based on the Dietary Guidelines for Americans (>100 mmol of sodium $\cong$ >2,400 mg sodium $\cong$ >6,000 mg of salt [sodium chloride per day]) (NCHS, 2008). Further, the Dietary Guidelines for Americans (HHS and USDA, 2005) and the AHA recommend that African Americans and persons who are middle aged or older or who have hypertension should consume less than 1,500 mg of sodium daily. Calculated sodium intake may not be accurate because the large majority of sodium in the U.S. food supply is added in processing and manufacturing of foods, and a large and increasing amount is used in the fast food industry. The amounts added can vary widely by brand and with time, making calculations difficult, and the smaller amounts added at home can also be challenging to quantify. Unfortunately, 24-hour urinary sodium excretion, which provides the best measure of sodium intake, has never been assessed in a nationally representative sample of the U.S. population, so that the true distribution of intakes in the United States is not known.

The committee finds the evidence base to support policies to reduce dietary sodium as a means to shift the population distribution of blood pressure levels in the population convincing. The newly reported analysis of the substantial health benefits (reduced number of individuals with hypertension) and the equally substantial health care cost savings and quality adjusted life years (QALYs) saved by reducing sodium intake to or below the recommended levels, provide resounding support to place a high priority on policies to reduce sodium intake (Palar and Sturm, 2009).

The committee is aware of the Congressional directive to the CDC to engage in activities to reduce sodium intake and the DHDSP's role in these activities. The DHDSP's sponsorship of an IOM study to identify a range of interventions to reduce dietary sodium intake is an important step. The committee believes that the DHDSP is well positioned to take greater leadership in this area through it role as co-leader of Healthy People 2010 Focus Area 12: Heart Disease and Stroke, co-leader of the National Forum for Heart Disease and Stroke Prevention, and as the sponsor of grants to state health departments and other entities.

4.4 The committee recommends that the Division for Heart Disease and Stroke Prevention take active leadership in convening other partners in federal, state, and local government and industry to advocate for and implement strategies to reduce sodium in the American diet to meet dietary guidelines, which are currently less than 2,300 mg/day (equivalent to 100 mmol/day) for the general population and 1,500 mg/day (equivalent to 70 mmol/day) for blacks, middle-aged and older adults, and individuals with hypertension.

The committee recognizes other work in progress by the IOM Committee on Strategies to Reduce Sodium Intake; therefore, it did not develop specific recommendations or specific intervention strategies.

Of all of the modifiable risk factors for hypertension, an inadequate consumption of potassium based on the current Dietary Reference Intake (DRI) criteria (IOM, 2004) is among the most prevalent. In a recent report from the CDC (NCHS, 2008), approximately 2 percent of U.S. adults met the current guidelines for dietary potassium intake (≥ 4.7 grams per day or 4,700 mg), but insufficient potassium intake is most prevalent in blacks and Hispanics, among whom the proportion consuming an adequate amount of potassium was close to 0 percent. Of note, the primary basis of the DRI of 4.7 grams per day for potassium is its beneficial effect on blood pressure (IOM, 2004).

4.5 The committee recommends that the Division for Heart Disease and Stroke Prevention specifically consider as a strategy advocating for the greater use of potassium/sodium chloride combinations as a means of simultaneously reducing sodium intake and increasing potassium intake.

State and local health jurisdictions can also play a strong role in formulating policies and other activities to reduce sodium in the diet. Across the country, 26 state and local public health agencies and 17 professional associations and organizations have coalesced to work toward the goal of reducing salt intake through the National Salt Reduction Initiative (The City of New York, 2009).

6.3 The committee recommends that all state and local public health jurisdictions immediately begin to consider developing a portfolio of dietary sodium reduction strategies that make the most sense for early action in their jurisdictions.

Surveillance

Data collection is fundamental to addressing any public health problem. Data are critical for determining the burden of hypertension, characterizing the patterns among subgroups of the population, assessing changes in the problem over time, and evaluating the success of interventions. Repeated independent cross-sectional surveys in the same populations over time can provide important information about secular trends in blood pressure. In the general U.S. population, government surveys (NHES I [National Health Examination Survey]; NHANES I, II, and III [National Health and Nutrition Examination Survey]; HHANES [Hispanic Health and Nutrition Examination Survey]) may provide the best data to examine secular trends in hypertension. However, there are marked, not easily explainable changes in the temporal trends for hypertension based on the NHANES data. In particular, there was a dramatic reduction in age-adjusted hypertension prevalence between the NHANES II (1976-1980) from 31.8 to 20 percent in the NHANES III (1988-1991). At the same time, there have been significant modifications in the protocol for blood pressure measurement, sample sizes, and other factors that may increase the potential for measurement error (Burt et al., 1995). As a consequence, there is ongoing uncertainty about the validity and therefore usefulness of long-term temporal data for U.S. trends in hypertension.

Effective monitoring and surveillance systems need to be in place to monitor progress in reducing the prevalence of hypertension and increasing the awareness, treatment, and control of hypertension. Given the challenges posed by the changing methodologies used to collect blood pressure measurements, the committee believes that efforts to strengthen hypertension surveillance and monitoring are critical.

2.1 The committee recommends that the Division for Heart Disease and Stroke Prevention

- Identify methods to better use (analyze and report) existing data on the monitoring and surveillance of hypertension over time.
- Develop norms for data collection, analysis, and reporting of future surveillance of blood pressure levels and hypertension.

In developing better data collection methods and analyses, the DHDSP should increase and improve analysis and reporting of understudied populations including: children, racial and ethnic minorities, the elderly, and socioeconomic groups.

Access to and use of hypertension measures at the state and local public health jurisdictions (SLHJs) level has proven especially difficult. The primary national data source for population estimates of hypertension—National Health and Nutrition Examination Survey—is not designed to produce accurate state or local estimates. This shortcoming is a major one, as there is likely substantial variation across regions not only in prevalence but also in the proportions of the hypertensive population not diagnosed, diagnosed but not under treatment, and under treatment but not controlled. Some state and localities have begun to develop local level HANES to better monitor hypertension.

6.4 The committee recommends that state and local public health jurisdictions assess their capacity to develop local HANES as a means to obtain local estimates of the prevalence, awareness, treatment, and control of hypertension. Further, if a program to reduce hypertension is a national goal, funding should be made available to assure that localities have relevant data that will assist them in addressing hypertension in their communities.

The committee recognizes that local financial constraints may not allow many SLHJs to move forward in this regard in the short term; thus, SLHJs may want to actively seek other reliable and available population-based data sets as a way to monitor local hypertension trends.

Accurate information on sodium intake or the content of sodium in specific foods that presently contribute importantly to sodium intake is necessary for monitoring its reduction. These data are not currently available in a systematic or timely fashion. The lack of data presents a significant gap that will hamper efforts to evaluate the progress made in reducing sodium intake in the American population.

4.6 The committee recommends that the Division for Heart Disease and Stroke Prevention and other CDC units explore methods to develop and implement data-gathering strategies that will allow for more accurate assessment and tracking of specific foods that are important contributors to dietary sodium intake by the American people.

4.7 The committee recommends that the Division for Heart Disease and Stroke Prevention and other CDC units explore methods to develop and implement data-gathering strategies that will allow for more accurate assessment and the tracking of population-level dietary sodium and potassium intake including the monitoring of 24-hour urinary sodium and potassium excretion.

System Change Strategies Directed at Individuals with Hypertension

Although patient nonadherence to treatment is one reason for lack of hypertension control, the lack of physician adherence to Joint National Committee on Prevention, Detection, Evaluation, and Treatment of High Blood Pressure guidelines (JNC) contributes to the lack of awareness, lack of pharmacologic and nonpharmacologic treatment, and lack of hypertension control in the United States (Chiong, 2008; Pavlik et al., 1997). Studies show that despite the JNC recommendation to screen and to start treatment if systolic blood pressure is >140 mm Hg or diastolic blood pressure is >90 mm Hg, physicians are not providing treatment consistent with the guidelines. In particular, physicians are less aggressive in treating elevated blood pressure in older patients and less aggressive in treating isolated systolic hypertension (Berlowitz et al., 1998; Chiong, 2008; Hyman et al., 2000; Izzo et al., 2000; Lloyd-Jones et al., 2002). In fact, the largest attributable fraction for lack of awareness and lack of control of hypertension is being aged 65 or older and having isolated hypertension. According to Hyman and Pavlik (2001), "Undiagnosed hypertension and treated but uncontrolled hypertension occurs largely under the watchful eye of the health care system." While the reasons for physician nonadherence to JNC guidelines are unclear, lack of physician awareness and physician beliefs about the practicality and benefit of treatment may contribute.

The goal of improving the education and training of health care providers in the prevention of cardiovascular disease is central to DHDSP activities. Numerous questions remain regarding whether the lack of adherence is related to a lack of physician agreement with the new treatment guidelines, physician lack of knowledge regarding the guidelines, inertia based on treating at the previous guideline of 160 mm Hg/95 mm Hg, or other barriers.

5.1 The committee recommends that the Division for Heart Disease and Stroke Prevention give high priority to conducting research to better understand the reasons behind poor physician adherence to current JNC guidelines. Once these factors are better understood, strategies should be developed to increase the likelihood that primary providers will screen for and treat hypertension appropriately, especially in elderly patients.

5.2 The committee recommends that the Division for Heart Disease and Stroke Prevention work with the Joint Commission and the health care quality community to improve provider performance on measures focused on assessing adherence to guidelines for screening for hypertension, the development of a hypertension disease management plan that is consistent with JNC guidelines, and achievement of blood pressure control.

6.5 The committee recommends that state and local public health jurisdictions serve as conveners of health care system representatives, physician groups, purchasers of health care services, quality improvement organizations, and employers (and others) to develop a plan to engage and leverage skills and resources for improving the medical treatment of hypertension.

Controlling for health status, financial burden has been shown to be significantly greater for persons with chronic conditions such as hypertension (Rogowski et al., 1997). Many studies, using a variety of methodologies, have documented a relationship between patient cost and poorer adherence to treatment and poorer control of hypertension (Fihn and Wicher, 1988). Out-of-pocket cost of medication has been identified in the literature as a significant barrier to patient adherence to hypertension treatment. It is estimated that for every 10 percent increase in cost-sharing, overall prescription drug spending decreases by 2-6 percent (Kilgore and Goldman, 2008). The impact of out-of-pocket costs is greatest for those with low income, those with chronic illnesses, and those taking multiple drugs (Austvoll-Dahlgren et al., 2008). Reducing out-of-pocket costs increases medication adherence. Goldman et al., (2007) compared the impact of reducing out-of-pocket costs with other interventions designed to improve patient adherence to chronic medications and noted that even the most successful interventions designed to increase patient adherence to medication did not result in larger improvements in adherence than cost strategies and generally relied on complicated, labor-intensive regimens. The committee finds the evidence convincing that reducing costs of antihypertensive medication is an important and efficient way to increase medication adherence.

> **5.3 The committee recommends that the Division for Heart Disease and Stroke Prevention should encourage the Centers for Medicare & Medicaid Services to recommend the elimination or reduction of deductibles for antihypertensive medications among plans participating under Medicare Part D, and work with state Medicaid programs and encourage them to eliminate deductibles and copayments for antihypertensive medications. The committee also recommends that the DHDSP work with the pharmaceutical industry and its trade organizations to standardize and simplify applications for patient assistance programs that provide reduced-cost or free antihypertensive medications for low-income, underinsured or uninsured individuals.**

> **6.6 State and local public health jurisdictions should work with business coalitions and purchasing coalitions to remove economic barriers to effective antihypertensive medications for individuals who have difficulty accessing them.**

The committee notes that the DHDSP is also well positioned to educate the private sector that eliminating or reducing the costs of antihypertensive medications is an important and efficient way to increase medication adherence. Through collaborations with partners, the DHDSP provides support and guidance to the employer community on hypertension and cardiovascular disease prevention and control. The private sector is already experimenting with reducing copayments associated with drugs commonly prescribed for diabetes, asthma, and hypertension (Pitney Bowes, Marriott, and others). The results of the studies showing the impact of cost-sharing and the reporting of improved outcomes from these company's experiences should be shared broadly with the business community through trade associations and purchasing coalitions.

> **5.4 The committee recommends that the Division for Heart Disease and Stroke Prevention collaborate with leaders in the business community to educate them about the impact of reduced patient costs on antihypertensive medication adherence and work with them to encourage employers to leverage their health care purchasing power to advocate for reduced deductibles and copayments for antihypertensive medications in their health insurance benefits packages.**

The use of community health workers to support the care of individuals with hypertension has been identified as a promising strategy. Community health workers have contributed to higher medication adherence among individuals with hypertension and have been shown to play an important role in linking and navigating diverse communities to the health care system. Some of the roles and the successes achieved appear to be similar to those of nurses who have provided educational interventions aimed at hypertension control, and suggest an efficient strategy for bringing about enhanced treatment and sustained blood pressure control for targeted racially or ethnically diverse, high-risk populations. While trained laypeople cannot perform in the same capacity as professional nurses and health educators, with appropriate training and supervision they can successfully contribute to the care of community members with hypertension (Bosworth et al., 2005).

Community health workers may also play an important role in linking diverse communities to the health care system (HRSA, 2007). The IOM committee that produced the report *Unequal Treatment: Confronting Racial and Ethnic Disparities in Healthcare* found that "community health workers offer promise as a community-based resource to increase racial and ethnic minorities' access to healthcare and to serve as a liaison between healthcare providers and the communities they serve." Based on this finding, the committee recommended supporting the use of community health workers. "Programs to support the use of community health workers (e.g., as health care navigators), especially among medically underserved and racial and ethnic minority populations, should be expanded, evaluated, and replicated" (IOM, 2003, p. 195).

5.5 The committee recommends that the Division for Heart Disease and Stroke Prevention work with state partners to leverage opportunities to ensure that existing community health worker programs include a focus on the prevention and control of hypertension. In the absence of such programs, the division should work with state partners to develop programs of community health workers who would be deployed in high-risk communities to help support healthy living strategies that include a focus on hypertension.

6.7 State and local public health jurisdictions should promote and work with community health worker initiatives to ensure that prevention and control of hypertension is included in the array of services they provide and are appropriately linked to primary care services.

In an era of declining resources and conflicting priorities for public health, taking on any new challenges needs careful consideration. But given the disease and economic burden associated with hypertension, and in the current climate of health care reform and increasing attention to prevention, there is great public health opportunity and no better time to rise to the challenge.

6.8 The committee recommends that Congress give priority to assuring adequate resources for implementing a broad suite of population-based policy and system approaches at the federal, state, and local levels that have the greatest promise to prevent, treat, and control hypertension.

Attendant to current funding and potential future funding for hypertension prevention, treatment, and control, systems need to be in place to track and measure current and new programs activities at the federal, state, and local level. Such a system would help ensure that resources are appropriately aligned and outcomes are achieved.

6.9 The committee recommends that the Division for Heart Disease and Stroke Prevention develop resource accountability systems to track and measure all current and new state programs for the prevention, treatment, and control of hypertension that would allow for resources to be assessed for alignment with the population-based policy and systems strategy and for measuring the outcomes achieved.

The committee acknowledges that the recommendations proffered, if adopted, would result in a significant programmatic change for the DHDSP. To effectively support the change and maintain a population-based focus, new expertise and guidance may be required beyond that which may be available through the DHDSP's partnership with the National Forum for Heart Disease and Stroke Prevention.

6.10 The committee recommends that the Division for Heart Disease and Stroke Prevention identify and work with experts grounded in population-based approaches to provide guidance and assistance in designing and executing hypertension prevention and control efforts that focus on population-based policy and system change. These experts could augment an existing advisory body or be drawn from an existing body with this expertise.

The committee believes that attention to the high-priority areas it has identified would ultimately lead to a reduction in the prevalence of hypertension, improve the quality of care provided to individuals with hypertension, reduce health disparities, and ultimately reduce mortality and morbidity due to heart disease and stroke.

In the short term, one visible impact would be strong federal, state, and local public health agency leadership that gives priority to reducing the prevalence of hypertension through population-based approaches integrated throughout agency activities, particularly those that target hypertension risk factors by reducing obesity, promoting healthy diets, increasing physical activity, and reducing sodium intake.

Active engagement and efforts by federal, state, and local jurisdiction to reduce sodium consumption, an area not typically addressed by parts of the governmental public health system, is an area where federal and SLHJs could exert a unique leadership role. Efforts to improve the surveillance and monitoring systems that track hypertension trends would result in improved estimates of hypertension prevalence, awareness, and treatment and control for the population as a whole and subgroups of the population at the national, state, and local levels. Similarly, with improved data collection, public health officials would be able to monitor their progress in reducing dietary sodium consumption and the sodium content in food. Strategies designed to address the factors contributing to poor physician adherence to JNC treatment guidelines would result in improved blood pressure control, especially isolated systolic hypertension among the elderly. The visible impacts of removing economic barriers to effective antihypertensive medications and employing the use of community health workers to provide community-based support for individuals with hypertension would be improved access to treatment, particularly for vulnerable populations.

The committee observes that hypertension may provide an opportunity unparalleled in public health chronic disease prevention for program evaluation through outcome measurement. In this context, it provides a single, reliable outcome measure that can be linked to intervention process measures to rapidly inform program interventions.

The committee offers a number of short-term and intermediate outcomes and potential process and outcome indicators to assess progress in the high-priority areas in Table S-2. Decreased mortality and morbidity from heart disease and stroke are understood as the ultimate long-term indicators, and as such, they are not included in the table due to space consideration. The table is divided into broad sections (e.g., Population-Based Recommendations to the DHDSP and SLHJs, System Approaches Targeting Individuals with Hypertension Directed to CDC and SLHJs, and others. Outcomes and indicators found in adjacent columns do not tract directly across but correspond to the group of recommendations.

TABLE S-2 Priority Recommendations

Population-Based Recommendations to the Division for Heart Disease and Stroke Prevention (DHDSP) and State and Local Public Health Jurisdictions (SLHJs)

Recommendations to Enhance Population-Based Efforts and to Strengthen Efforts Among CDC Units and Partners

Priority Recommendation	Short-Term Outcomes (or process input or outputs)	Short-Term Indicator	Intermediate Outcomes	Intermediate Indicators
4.1 The DHDSP should integrate hypertension prevention and control in programmatic efforts to effect system, environmental, and policy changes through collaboration with other CDC units and their external partners. High-priority programmatic activities on which to collaborate include interventions for: -reducing overweight and obesity, -promoting the consumption of a healthy diet, -increasing potassium-rich fruits and vegetables in the diet, and -increasing physical activity.	Better targeting and integration of hypertension prevention in other CDC unit programming	Budget allocated to population-based policy and system approaches by the CDC	Reduction of hypertension risk factors in the population	Prevalence of overweight/obesity Proportion of individuals who consume a healthy diet
4.2 Population-based interventions to improve physical activity and food environments (typically the focus of other CDC units) should include an evaluation of their feasibility and effectiveness, and their specific impact on hypertension prevalence and control.	New CDC budget and programs dedicated to policy and program system change strategies for hypertension Greater collaboration among CDC units on population-based interventions to prevent hypertension	Budget and plans for hypertension program integration into other CDC prevention activities Number of CDC activities that include a focus on hypertension prevention and control	Reduced incidence of hypertension Data on feasibility and effectiveness of a broad range of interventions that contribute to the prevention of hypertension	Proportion of children and adults who participate regularly in physical activities Reduction in adverse lifestyle behaviors

Recommendation		Indicator	Intermediate Outcome	Long-term Outcome
4.3 The DHDSP should leverage its ability to shape state activities, through its grant making and cooperative agreements, to encourage state activities to shift toward population-based prevention of hypertension.	Prevention of hypertension integrated in other unit strategies to: reduce overweight and obesity, promote healthy diet, increase consumption of fruits and vegetables, increase physical activity	Number of federal, state, and community policy and environmental strategies implemented to control high blood pressure	Reduced prevalence of hypertension	Percent reduction in disparities in high blood pressure risk factors between general and priority populations
6.1 SLHJs should give priority to population-based approaches over individual-based approaches to prevent and control hypertension.		Number of SLHJs that have added hypertension program elements and focus to nonhypertension programs		
6.2 SLHJs should integrate hypertension prevention and control in programmatic efforts to effect system, environmental, and policy changes that will support healthy eating, active living, and obesity prevention. Existing and new programmatic efforts should be assessed to ensure they are aligned with populations, most likely to be affected by hypertension such as older populations, which are often not the target of these programs.	Strong federal, state, and local public health agency leadership that gives priority to reducing the prevalence of hypertension through population-based approaches integrated throughout agency activities	Number of SLHJs with comprehensive programs for population hypertension control programs		

continued

TABLE S-2 Continued

Recommendations to Strengthen Leadership in Reducing Sodium Intake and Increasing Potassium Intake

Priority Recommendation	Short-Term Outcomes (or process input or outputs)	Short-Term Indicator	Intermediate Outcomes	Intermediate Indicators
4.4 The DHDSP should take active leadership in convening other partners in federal, state, and local government and industry to advocate for and implement strategies to reduce sodium in the American diet to meet dietary guidelines, which are currently less than 2,300 mg/day (equivalent to 100 mmol/day) for the general population and 1,500 mg/day (equivalent to 70 mmol/day) for blacks, middle-aged and older adults, and individuals with hypertension.	Aggressive actions at the federal, state, and local levels to reduce sodium consumption and sodium content in the diet Development and implementation of federal, state, land ocal programs to reduce sodium intake	Proportion of states and localities with a strategic plan to reduce sodium intake and sodium content in food Federal, state, and local budgets and plans for programs to reduce sodium intake	Reduction of salt consumption by the American population Reduction of salt content in food Reduced prevalence of hypertension	Mean population urinary sodium excretion level Proportion of individuals who consume five or more fruits and vegetables per day

6.3 SLHJs should immediately begin to consider developing a portfolio of dietary sodium reduction strategies that make the most sense for early action in their jurisdictions.	Number of states implementing new or expanded programs to increase potassium rich fruit and vegetable consumption			Mean population urinary potassium excretion level
4.5 DHDSP should specifically consider as a strategy advocating for the greater use of potassium/sodium chloride combinations as a means of simultaneously reducing sodium intake and increasing potassium intake.	Development and implementation of programs to increase potassium intake	Budget and plans for programs for increasing potassium consumption	Increase in potassium rich fruit and vegetable consumption Reduction of hypertension risk factors in the population	Mean and median blood pressure levels

continued

TABLE S-2 Continued

Recommendations to Improve the Surveillance and Reporting of Hypertension and Risk Factors

Priority Recommendation	Short-Term Outcomes (or process input or outputs)	Short-Term Indicator	Intermediate Outcomes	Intermediate Indicators
2.1 The DHDSP should identify methods to better use (analyze and report) existing data on the monitoring and surveillance of hypertension over time and develop norms for data collection, analysis, and reporting of future surveillance of blood pressure levels and hypertension. In developing better data collection methods and analyses, the DHDSP should increase and improve analysis and reporting of understudied populations including: children, racial and ethnic minorities, the elderly, and socioeconomic groups.	Guidance on methods for analyzing and reporting existing data for monitoring and surveillance of hypertension and future data collection methods and analyses	Improved estimates of hypertension prevalence, awareness, treatment, and control for the population as a whole and subgroups of the population (children, racial and ethnic minorities, the elderly, and socioeconomic groups) at the national, state, and local levels	Improved capacity for assessing and monitoring progress in hypertension prevention and control	Improved program design and implementation as a result of better data
6.4 SLHJs should assess their capacity to develop local HANES as a means to obtain local estimates of the prevalence, awareness, treatment, and control of hypertension. Further, if a program to reduce hypertension is a national goal, funding should be made available to assure that localities have relevant data that will assist them in addressing hypertension in their communities.	Increased number of state and localities with a NHANES-like survey	Number of states and localities with data systems that provide estimates of the prevalence, awareness, treatment, and control of hypertension for their jurisdictions	Access to local data on hypertension trends	Number of states and localities that are implementing program changes based on local surveillance and reporting information

4.6 The DHDSP and other CDC units, should explore methods to develop and implement data-gathering strategies that will allow for more accurate assessment and tracking of specific foods that are important contributors to dietary sodium intake by the American people.	Improved systems for measuring or estimating sodium content in food are designed and implemented	Availability of data on specific foods that are important contributors to dietary sodium intake by the American people	Data on high-sodium-containing foods are tracked and used to develop strategies for reduction	Percent of high content sodium products that have reduced their sodium content
4.7 The DHDSP and other CDC units should explore methods to develop and implement data-gathering strategies that will allow for more accurate assessment and the tracking of population-level dietary sodium and potassium intake including the monitoring of 24-hour urinary sodium and potassium excretion.	Improved systems for measuring or estimating dietary sodium and potassium intake are designed and implemented	Availability of mean population dietary sodium and potassium intake at the national, state, and local levels	Data on dietary sodium consumption are available and used to target dietary sodium reduction programs	Reduction in mean dietary sodium intake

continued

TABLE S-2 Continued

System Change Recommendations Directed at Individuals with Hypertension

Recommendations to Improve the Quality of Care Provided to Individuals with Hypertension

Priority Recommendation	Short-Term Outcomes (or process input or outputs)	Short-Term Indicator	Intermediate Outcomes	Intermediate Indicators
5.1 The DHDSP should give high priority to conducting research to better understand the reasons behind poor physician adherence to current JNC guidelines. Once these factors are better understood, strategies should be developed to increase the likelihood that primary providers will screen for and treat hypertension appropriately, especially in elderly patients.	Better understanding of reasons behind poor physician adherence to JNC guidelines Targeted strategies to improve provider awareness, understanding, acceptance, and adherence to JNC treatment guidelines	Proportion of providers who measure and classify blood pressure according to JNC guidelines Proportion of providers who follow JNC pharmacologic therapies for treatment of hypertension	Improved rates of diagnosed, treated, and controlled patients, especially systolic blood pressure control among the elderly	Proportion of individuals with hypertension who have achieved blood pressure control

5.2 The DHDSP should work with The Joint Commission and the health care quality community to improve provider performance on measures focused on assessing adherence to guidelines for screening for hypertension, the development of a hypertension disease management plan that is consistent with JNC guidelines, and achievement of blood pressure control.	Partnerships with health care quality community focused on improving provider performance on quality measure for hypertension	Proportion of patients who receive provider-initiated prescription and follow-up of therapeutic lifestyle modifications Proportion of patients with uncontrolled high blood pressure who have documented provider initiated change in pharmaceutical intervention	Improvements in state- or local-level provider performance in quality measures associated with blood pressure treatment and control	Proportion of older individuals with systolic hypertension who receive appropriate treatment
6.5 SLHJs should serve as conveners of health care system representatives, physician groups, purchasers of health care services, quality improvement organizations, and employers (and others) to develop a plan to engage and leverage skills and resources for improving the medical treatment of hypertension.	Development of local-level partnerships between SLHJs and health care representatives, physician groups, purchasers of health care services, quality improvement organizations, and employers around hypertension prevention and control	Development of local collaborative plans to address hypertension prevention, control, and treatment		Improvement in state reported diagnosis, treatment, and control rates

continued

TABLE S-2 Continued

Recommendations to Remove Economic Barriers to Effective Antihypertensive Medications

Priority Recommendation	Short-Term Outcomes (or process input or outputs)	Short-Term Indicator	Intermediate Outcomes	Intermediate Indicators
5.3 The DHDSP should encourage the Centers for Medicare & Medicaid Services to recommend the elimination or reduction of deductibles for antihypertensive medications among plans participating under Medicare Part D, and work with state Medicaid programs and encourage them to eliminate deductibles and copayments for antihypertensive medications. The DHDSP should work with the pharmaceutical industry and its trade organizations to standardize and simplify applications for patient assistance programs that provide reduced-cost or free antihypertensive medications for low-income, underinsured, or uninsured individuals.	Reduced cost for effective antihypertensive medication, especially among the poor, elderly, and those without health insurance coverage	Out-of-pocket costs for antihypertensive medications by insurance and economic status	Improved adherence to antihypertensive medications especially in the poor, elderly, and those without health insurance coverage Improved hypertension control, especially in the poor, elderly, and those without health insurance coverage	Prevalence of controlled hypertension, especially in the poor, elderly, and those without health insurance coverage Proportion of patients who adhere to antihypertensive medication regimens Degree of disparity in blood pressure control between general and priority populations

5.4 The DHDSP should collaborate with leaders in the business community to educate them about the impact of reduced patient costs on antihypertensive medication adherence and work with them to encourage employers to leverage their health care purchasing power to advocate for reduced deductibles and copayments for antihypertensive medications in their health insurance benefits packages.	Partnerships between the DHDSP and business community focused on reducing out-of-pocket costs for antihypertensive medications	Out-of-pocket costs for antihypertensive medications for worksite employees	Improved adherence to antihypertensive medications among employees	Proportion of employees who adhere to antihypertensive medication regimens

Degree of disparity in blood pressure control between general and priority employee populations |
| 6.6 SLHJs should work with business coalitions and purchasing coalitions to remove economic barriers to effective antihypertensive medications for individuals who have difficulty accessing them. | Partnerships between SLHJs and business community focused on reducing out-of-pocket costs for antihypertensive medications | | | |

continued

TABLE S-2 Continued

Recommendations to Provide Community Support for Individuals with Hypertension

Priority Recommendation	Short-Term Outcomes (or process input or outputs)	Short-Term Indicator	Intermediate Outcomes	Intermediate Indicators
5.5 The DHDSP should work with state partners to leverage opportunities to ensure that existing community health worker programs include a focus on the prevention and control of hypertension. In the absence of such programs, the DHDSP should work with state partners to develop programs of community health workers who would be deployed in high-risk communities to help support healthy living strategies that include a focus on hypertension.	Design and implementation of new or enhanced community health worker programs targeting hypertension control	Budget allocated to development or enhancement of community health worker programs Number of community health worker programs targeting hypertension	Improved hypertension control in communities served by community health worker programs	Prevalence of uncontrolled hypertension in communities served by community health workers Degree of reduction in disparities in blood pressure control between general population and populations served by community health workers
6.7 SLHJs should promote and work with community health worker initiatives to ensure that prevention and control of hypertension is included in the array of services they provide and are appropriately linked to primary care services.				

Hypertension as a Sentinel Indicator for Health Disparities

Hypertension is a disease for which there are major inequities across racial groups and economic groups—along the entire spectrum from risk factors to delivery of medical care. Interventions directed toward general population groups historically do not correct these inequities and can even worsen them. Care must be taken to assure that any portfolio of interventions implemented will minimize existing inequities in prevention, detection, treatment, and control of hypertension.

Hypertension is a condition strongly influenced by underlying individual and community risk factors related to healthy eating and active living—risk factors driven by race and class in most communities today. As such, it is a potential sentinel indicator for assessing and testing broader approaches to reduce health disparities. The prevalence of hypertension may provide a relatively quick and objective measure of programs directed at these risk factors as well as underlying social determinants of health. Hypertension, while treatable, requires ongoing access to primary care for maximum effectiveness. As such, it is also a potentially very good marker for lack of access to or continuity of health care in a community. SLHJs should consider hypertension as a sentinel measure for evaluation of the effectiveness of a range of disparity-reducing activities, including important place-based strategies tackling conditions through community policy interventions.

REFERENCES

Austvoll-Dahlgren, A., M. Aaserud, G. Vist, C. Ramsay, A. D. Oxman, H. Sturm, J. P. Kosters, and A. Vernby. 2008. Pharmaceutical policies: Effects of cap and co-payment on rational drug use. *Cochrane Database of Systematic Reviews* (1).

Baker, E. L., and J. Porter. 2005. Practicing management and leadership: Creating the information network for public health officials. *Journal of Public Health Management and Practice* 11(5):469-473.

Balu, S., and J. Thomas, 3rd. 2006. Incremental expenditure of treating hypertension in the United States. *American Journal of Hypertension* 19(8):810-816.

Berlowitz, D. R., A. S. Ash, E. C. Hickey, R. H. Friedman, M. Glickman, B. Kader, and M. A. Moskowitz. 1998. Inadequate management of blood pressure in a hypertensive population. *New England Journal of Medicine* 339(27):1957-1963.

Bosworth, H. B., M. K. Olsen, P. Gentry, M. Orr, T. Dudley, F. McCant, and E. Z. Oddone. 2005. Nurse administered telephone intervention for blood pressure control: A patient-tailored multifactorial intervention. *Patient Education and Counseling* 57(1):5-14.

Burt, V. L., J. A. Cutler, M. Higgins, M. J. Horan, D. Labarthe, P. Whelton, C. Brown, and E. J. Roccella. 1995. Trends in the prevalence, awareness, treatment, and control of hypertension in the adult US population. Data from the health examination surveys, 1960 to 1991. *Hypertension* 26(1):60-69.

CDC (Centers for Disease Control and Prevention). 2006. *Healthy People 2010 Midcourse Review: Section 12: Heart disease and stroke.* http://www.healthypeople.gov/data/midcourse/pdf/fa12.pdf (accessed February 4, 2010).

Chiong, J. R. 2008. Controlling hypertension from a public health perspective. *International Journal of Cardiology* 127(2):151-156.

Chobanian, A. V., G. L. Bakris, H. R. Black, W. C. Cushman, L. A. Green, J. L. Izzo, Jr., D. W. Jones, B. J. Materson, S. Oparil, J. T. Wright, Jr., and E. J. Roccella. 2003. The Seventh Report of the Joint National Committee on Prevention, Detection, Evaluation, and Treatment of High Blood Pressure: The JNC 7 Report. *Journal of the American Medical Association* 289(19):2560-2572.

Cutler, D. M., G. Long, E. R. Berndt, J. Royer, A. A. Fournier, A. Sasser, and P. Cremieux. 2007. The value of antihypertensive drugs: A perspective on medical innovation. *Health Affairs* 26(1):97-110.

DeVol, R., and A. Bedroussian. 2007. *An unhealthy America: The economic burden of chronic disease.* Santa Monica, CA: Milken Institute.

Fields, L. E., V. L. Burt, J. A. Cutler, J. Hughes, E. J. Roccella, and P. Sorlie. 2004. The burden of adult hypertension in the United States 1999 to 2000: A rising tide. *Hypertension* 44(4):398-404.

Fihn, S. D., and J. B. Wicher. 1988. Withdrawing routine outpatient medical services: Effects on access and health. *Journal of General Internal Medicine* 3(4):356-362.

Goldman, D. P., G. F. Joyce, and Y. Zheng. 2007. Prescription drug cost sharing: Associations with medication and medical utilization and spending and health. *Journal of the American Medical Association* 298(1):61-69.

HHS (U.S. Department of Health and Human Services) and USDA (U.S. Department of Agriculture). *Dietary Guidelines for Americans, 2005.* 6th Edition. Washington, DC: U.S. Government Printing Office.

HRSA (Health Resources and Services Adminstration). 2007. *Community health workers national workforce study.* Washington, DC: U.S. Department of Health and Human Services.

Hyman, D. J., and V. N. Pavlik. 2001. Characteristics of patients with uncontrolled hypertension in the United States. [see comment] [erratum appears in 2002 *New England Journal of Medicine* 346(7):544]. *New England Journal of Medicine* 345(7):479-486.

Hyman, D. J., V. N. Pavlik, and C. Vallbona. 2000. Physician role in lack of awareness and control of hypertension. *Journal of Clinical Hypertension (Greenwich)* 2(5):324-330.

IOM (Institute of Medicine). 2003. *Unequal treatment: Confronting racial and ethnic disparities in health care.* Washington, DC: The National Academies Press.

———. 2004. *Dietary reference intakes: Water, potassium, sodium, chloride, and sulfate.* Washington, DC: The National Academies Press.

Izzo, J. L., Jr., D. Levy, and H. R. Black. 2000. Clinical advisory statement. Importance of systolic blood pressure in older Americans. *Hypertension* 35(5):1021-1024.

Kilgore, M. L., and D. P. Goldman. 2008. Drug costs and out-of-pocket spending in cancer clinical trials. *Contemporary Clinical Trials* 29(1):1-8.

Lloyd-Jones, D. M., J. C. Evans, M. G. Larson, and D. Levy. 2002. Treatment and control of hypertension in the community: A prospective analysis. *Hypertension* 40(5):640-646.

Lloyd-Jones, D., R. Adams, M. Carnethon, G. De Simone, T. B. Ferguson, K. Flegal, E. Ford, K. Furie, A. Go, K. Greenlund, N. Haase, S. Hailpern, M. Ho, V. Howard, B. Kissela, S. Kittner, D. Lackland, L. Lisabeth, A. Marelli, M. McDermott, J. Meigs, D. Mozaffarian, G. Nichol, C. O'Donnell, V. Roger, W. Rosamond, R. Sacco, P. Sorlie, R. Stafford, J. Steinberger, T. Thom, S. Wasserthiel-Smoller, N. Wong, J. Wylie-Rosett, and Y. Hong. 2009. Heart disease and stroke statistics—2009 update: A report from the American Heart Association Statistics Committee and Stroke Statistics Subcommittee. *Circulation* 119(3):480-486.

NCHS (National Center for Health Statistics). 2008. Healthy People 2010 progress review: Focus area 19: Nutrition and overweight presentation. http://www.cdc.gov/nchs/ppt/hp2010/focus_areas/fa19_2_ppt/fa19_nutrition2_ppt. htm (accessed September 14, 2009).

Palar, K., and R. Sturm. 2009. Potential societal savings from reduced sodium consumption in the U.S. adult population. *American Journal of Health Promotion* 24(1):49-57.

Pavlik, V. N., D. J. Hyman, C. Vallbona, C. Toronjo, and K. Louis. 1997. Hypertension awareness and control in an inner-city African-American sample. *Journal of Human Hypertension* 11(5):277-283.

Rogowski, J., L. A. Lillard, and R. Kington. 1997. The financial burden of prescription drug use among elderly persons. *Gerontologist* 37(4):475-482.

The City of New York. 2009. *Statement of commitment by health organizations and public agencies*. http://www.nyc.gov/html/doh/html/cardio/cardio-salt-coalition.shtml (accessed December 18, 2009).

Vasan, R. S., A. Beiser, S. Seshadri, M. G. Larson, W. B. Kannel, R. B. D'Agostino, and D. Levy. 2002. Residual lifetime risk for developing hypertension in middle-aged women and men: The Framingham Heart Study. *Journal of the American Medical Association* 287(8):1003-1010.

1

Introduction

In today's public health world, the term "neglected disease" conjures up obscure tropical illnesses of little relevance to contemporary practice in the United States. Yet, when one considers the actual meaning of the words, the time may be right to add hypertension to this list. Hypertension, or high blood pressure, describes the condition in which systemic arterial blood pressure remains elevated over time. High blood pressure is caused primarily by an increase in the resistance to the flow of blood through arteries and an increase in cardiac output, which is a function of the heart rate and stroke volume. Hypertension is dangerous because it forces the heart to work harder and can contribute to atherosclerosis and hardening of the large arteries causing cardiovascular disease. These factors can also lead to subsequent blockage and weakening of the walls of the smaller cerebral arteries causing them to rupture and result in stroke. The lack of attention to hypertension is difficult to understand. Hypertension is one of the leading causes of preventable death in the United States. A recent study (Danaei et al., 2009) listed it at number two, just behind tobacco. Based on data from the Centers for Disease Control and Prevention (CDC) and the National Heart, Lung, and Blood Institute (NHLBI) from 1995 to 2005, the death rate from high blood pressure increased by 25.2 percent and the actual number of deaths rose by 56.4 percent (Lloyd-Jones et al., 2009). In 2005, high blood pressure was responsible for about one in six deaths of U.S. adults. Further, high blood pressure is the single largest risk factor for cardiovascular mortality accounting for about 45 percent of all cardiovascular deaths. High blood pressure was the leading cause of death among women, accounting for 19 percent of all female deaths, and the second leading cause of death among men (second to smoking) (Lloyd-Jones et al., 2009). Hypertension is estimated to contribute to 35 percent of myocardial infarctions and strokes and 49 percent of episodes of heart failure (AHRQ, 2007).

Hypertension is diagnosed by a simple test. Using a sphygmomanometer, blood pressure is typically measured at two points: at peak pressure when the heart is most contracted (this point is referred to as systolic blood pressure) and then when the heart is most relaxed (diastolic pressure). High blood pressure for adults is defined as a systolic pressure of 140 mm Hg or greater or a diastolic pressure of 90 mm Hg or greater or using antihypertensive medication. Using this definition, hypertension is highly prevalent; nearly one in three U.S. adults has hypertension (Fields et al., 2004; Lloyd-Jones et al., 2009). The risk of developing hypertension increases with age. In older age groups it is more common than not; based on data from the Framingham study, the lifetime risk of hypertension is estimated to be 90 percent for people with normal blood pressure at age 55 or 65 who live to be age 80-85, respectively (Cutler et al., 2007; Vasan et al., 2002). Approximately 73 million Americans have high blood pressure, and an additional 59 million have prehypertension, which is defined as blood pressure ranging from 120-139 mm Hg systolic and/or 80-89 mm Hg diastolic. Prehypertension is a new classification introduced by the *Seventh Report of the Joint National Committee on Prevention, Detection, Evaluation, and Treatment of High Blood Pressure* (Chobanian et al., 2003)[1] because of the increasing amount of data associating cardiovascular complications with what had previously been considered normal blood pressure readings. Figure 1-1 shows the increased risk of heart disease death, and Figure 1-2 shows the increased risk of stroke death, associated with prehypertension and hypertension by decade of life. Starting at a systolic blood pressure of 115 mm Hg, every 20 mm Hg increase in systolic blood pressure is associated with a doubling in the risk of death from both heart disease and from stroke.

Hypertension is highly treatable, and a range of medications—some relatively inexpensive—are available. In the late 1950s and early 1960s, oral diuretics were primarily used to treat hypertension. Since then, additional medications including calcium channel blockers and beta-blockers, angiotensin-converting enzyme (ACE) inhibitors, and angiotensin receptor antagonists can be found among the antihypertensive therapies available

---

[1] The NHLBI administers the National High Blood Pressure Education Program Coordinating Committee, a coalition of 39 major professional, public, and voluntary organizations and 7 federal agencies. An important function of the committee is to issue guidelines and advisories designed to increase awareness, prevention, treatment, and control of hypertension. Reports from this body are referred to by their number: in this case, the *Seventh Report of the Joint National Committee on Prevention, Detection, Evaluation, and Treatment of High Blood Pressure* (Chobanian et al., 2003).

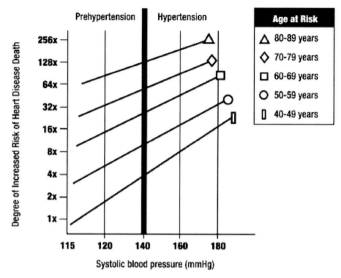

FIGURE 1-1 Increased risk of death from heart disease associated with blood pressure by decade of life.
SOURCE: NHLBI, 2004a.

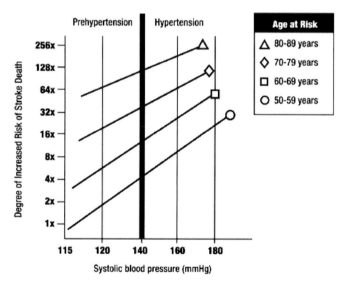

FIGURE 1-2 Increased risk of death from stroke associated with blood pressure by decade of life.
SOURCE: NHLBI, 2004a.

to physicians for managing high blood pressure. Studies comparing the effectiveness of antihypertensive therapies suggest that generally low-dose diuretics, which also tend to be lowest in cost,[2] are the most effective first line of treatment for preventing mortality and morbidity from cardiovascular disease (ALLHAT, 2002; Psaty et al., 2002).

More importantly, hypertension is highly preventable through a decrease in obesity, increase in physical activity, and improved diet (particularly through reduced sodium and increases in fruit and vegetable consumption). Moreover, since poor diet, physical inactivity, and obesity appear to be on the increase, reductions in these risk factors takes on even greater importance.

Finally, hypertension is costly to the healthcare system. It is the most common primary diagnosis in America (Chobanian et al., 2003), and it contributes to the costs of cardiovascular disease (coronary heart disease, myocardial infarction) and stroke. The methodologies used to estimate the costs associated with hypertension vary; one estimate reports the total economic burden of coronary heart disease and stroke as $120.6 billion and $48.9 billion, respectively, in 2002 (Cutler et al., 2007). The American Heart Association (AHA) recently reported the direct and indirect costs specifically of high blood pressure as a primary diagnosis as $73.4 billion for 2009 (Lloyd-Jones et al., 2009). With respect to the cost of treating hypertension, an analysis by DeVol and Bedroussian (2007) estimated that the total expenditure for the population reporting hypertension as a condition in the Medical Expenditure Panel Survey (MEPS) was $32.5 billion in 2003. Another study estimated the total incremental annual direct expenditures for treating hypertension (the excess expenditure of treating patients with hypertension compared to patients without hypertension) to be about $55 billion in 2001 (Balu and Thomas, 2006). More specifically, it is estimated that a 10 percent decrease in annual health care visits for hypertension would save $450 million each year in health care costs (NHLBI, 2004b).

CDC EFFORTS TO REDUCE AND CONTROL HYPERTENSION

The CDC is the lead federal agency responsible for promoting health and quality of life by preventing and controlling disease, injury, and disability. The CDC Division for Heart Disease and Stroke Prevention (DHDSP) provides national leadership to reduce the burden of disease, disability,

---

[2] A review of data from the Medical Expenditure Panel Survey (MEPS) analyzing trends in the pharmaceutical treatment of hypertension from 1977 to 2003 found that in 2003, diuretics were the most inexpensive antihypertensive drugs, with an average per user expenditure of $92 compared to calcium channel blockers with an average per user expenditure of $421 (Miller and Zodet, 2006).

and death from heart disease and stroke. DHDSP has six programmatic priority areas: (1) control high blood pressure, (2) control high cholesterol, (3) improve emergency response, (4) improve quality of care, (5) increase awareness of the signs and symptoms of heart attack and stroke and of the need to call 911, and (6) eliminate health disparities related to heart disease and stroke. The DHDSP carries out its programmatic responsibilities with a budget of $54 million for fiscal year 2009.

The DHDSP is co-lead, along with the NHLBI, for the Healthy People 2010 Focus Area 12 objectives related to heart disease and stroke including four objectives specific to hypertension (Table 1-1).

Findings from the Healthy People 2010 Midcourse Review (CDC, 2006) indicated that the nation was moving away from making progress in the target objectives as reflected by increases in the prevalence of high blood pressure among adults and among children and adolescents. This moving away from Healthy People 2010 goals provided an increased emphasis for a DHDSP programmatic focus on hypertension.

The DHDSP has developed a strategic plan to reduce and control hypertension that recognizes the urgent need to implement a number of effective practices and to develop new public health practices. The plan identifies a number of action areas and goals for the prevention and control of hypertension from which the most important priorities must be selected. These priorities must also take into consideration state health departments and other critical partners. The CDC requested assistance and guidance from the Institute of Medicine (IOM) to determine a small set of high-priority areas in which public health can focus its efforts to accelerate progress in hypertension reduction and control. Specifically, the CDC requested that

TABLE 1-1 Healthy People 2010 Focus Area 12: Heart and Stroke, Blood Pressure Objectives

Number	Objective
12-9.	Reduce the proportion of adults with high blood pressure.
12-10.	Increase the proportion of adults with high blood pressure whose blood pressure is under control.
12-11.	Increase the proportion of adults with high blood pressure who are taking action (for example, losing weight, increasing physical activity, or reducing sodium intake) to help control their blood pressure.
12-12.	Increase the proportion of adults who have had their blood pressure measured within the preceding 2 years and can state whether their blood pressure was normal or high.

SOURCE: CDC, 2006.

the IOM convene an expert committee to review available public health strategies for reducing and controlling hypertension in the U.S. population, including both science-based and practice-based knowledge. In conducting its work, the committee was asked to consider the following questions:

What are the highest-priority action areas on which the CDC's Division for Heart Disease and Stroke Prevention and other partners should focus near-term efforts in hypertension?

1   Identify the particular role of the CDC's DHDSP in addressing the highest-priority areas.
2. Identify the role of state health departments in advancing progress in the priority action areas.
3. Identify the role of other public health partners.
4. What visible impacts can be expected if the DHDSP focuses its efforts in these priority areas?
5. What indicators should be monitored to assess the progress of the DHDSP, state health departments, and partners in implementing the committee's recommendations?
6. What are the potential positive and negative impacts on health disparities that could result if the committee's recommendations are implemented?
7. What indicators should be monitored related to health disparities to ensure the intended impact of the DHDSP priority action areas identified?

The committee was not expected to conduct a new, detailed review of peer-reviewed literature on hypertension because such literature reviews, meta-analyses, and syntheses already exist and have been used to inform existing guidelines and recommendations.

The report is organized into six chapters, including this introduction, which discusses the study process and the committee's approach to questions it was asked to address. Chapter 2 provides a discussion of the public health importance of hypertension and an overview of hypertension trends in the United States. Chapter 3 provides an overview of the CDC's Division for Heart Disease and Stroke Prevention and background information on its budget and activities. Chapters 4 and 5 provide the committee's response to the task of identifying a small set of priority areas for the DHDSP in which public health can focus its efforts to accelerate progress in hypertension reduction and control. Specifically, Chapter 4 addresses priority areas for interventions that are directed at population-based risk factors that are known to increase the risk of hypertension in the general population. Chapter 5 addresses priority areas for interventions directed at individuals with hypertension. The recommendations in Chapters 4 and 5 are specifically directed to the DHDSP. The committee recognizes that the DHDSP cannot work in isolation to implement the population-based policy and system change approach to prevent and control hypertension; thus, it notes when partnerships with other partners are appropriate (for example the business community, health care quality community, and the Centers for Medicare & Medicaid Services). The committee, however, views state and local health jurisdictions to be critical DHDSP partners. In Chapter 6, the committee specifically recommends the action steps state and local health jurisdictions can take to implement the priority actions (response to question 2). Chapter 6 also provides the potential short-term and intermediate outcomes and potential indicators to be monitored to assess the progress made in implementing the committee's recommendations (questions 4 and 5). Because the committee's recommendations are population-based policy and system changes, it is expected that they could improve hypertension prevention, treatment, and control across all population and subgroups. However, the committee also argues that hypertension is a sentinel indicator for how well the public health system is reducing health disparities (racial and ethnic, age, geographic). Chapter 6 briefly comments on the potential positive and negative impacts on health disparities (questions 6 and 7).

Much is known about the health consequences and costs associated with hypertension. Robust clinical and public health research efforts have developed safe and cost-effective nonpharmacological and pharmacological interventions (Chapters 4 and 5) to prevent, treat, and control hypertension. Nonetheless, millions of Americans continue to develop, live with, and die from hypertension because we are failing to translate our public health and clinical knowledge into effective prevention, treatment, and control programs. In the committee's view this current state is one of neglect, defined by *Merriam-Webster* as "giving insufficient attention to something that merits attention." The recommendations offered in this report outline a population-based policy and systems change approach to addressing hypertension that can be applied at the federal, state, and local levels. It is time to give full attention and take concerted actions to prevent and control hypertension.

STUDY PROCESS

In response to the study request, the IOM established the Committee on Public Health Priorities to Reduce and Control Hypertension in the U.S. Population. The committee comprised experts from the areas of public health, prevention, epidemiology, health care, hypertension, cardiovascular disease, health disparities, and community-based interventions. (See Appendix A for biographies of the committee members.)

During the course of the study, the committee gathered information to address its charge through a variety of means. It conducted a review of pertinent literature and held three in-person information-gathering meetings with sessions that were open to the public. The first meeting included presentations from the sponsor and hypertension experts. The committee also received input on hypertension prevention and control strategies from representatives of a number of state, local, and nongovernmental agencies. The second meeting focused on learning more about the CDC Division for Heart Disease and Stroke Prevention's activities and reviewing data on blood pressure trends. At that meeting the committee also received information on the lessons learned from the National High Blood Pressure Education Program, the Hypertension Detection and Follow-up Program, and the Antihypertensive and Lipid-Lowering Treatment to Prevent Heart Attack Trial (ALLHAT) sponsored by the National Institutes of Health. The third meeting included presentations on health disparities in hypertension; past large-scale community-based interventions; and the effectiveness, cost, and coverage of hypertension interventions. Appendix B contains the agendas for public meetings. The committee also met in executive session for deliberative discussions following the information-gathering meetings.

Two additional meetings with open public sessions were held via teleconference calls. These sessions included presentations to the committee on blood pressure trends in birth cohorts, dietary interventions to reduce hypertension, the experiences of one State Heart Disease and Stroke Prevention Program, and specific aspects of the CDC's Heart Disease and Stroke Prevention Program. In addition to these meetings, the committee held conference calls to further discuss findings and to formulate recommendations.

STUDY APPROACH

The overall public health impact of high blood pressure is a function of the distribution of blood pressure in the population as well as the outcomes or health consequences of high blood pressure. Because of the continuous and graded relationship between blood pressure and adverse health outcomes, the committee supports the notion that public health efforts to prevent the health consequences of high blood pressure must consider not only reducing blood pressure among those with high levels but also shifting the distribution of blood pressure in the population as a whole (Ahern et al., 2008; Rose, 2001; Whelton et al., 2002). The committee also decided that a framework would be useful in the process of identifying potential priority public health strategies to reduce and control hypertension. The following section provides the framework used by the committee and the selection criteria considered in identifying potential priority strategies.

The population distribution of blood pressure and the health consequences of high blood pressure are the end results of a complex set of processes involving the action of factors at multiple levels ranging from macro-level and societal factors (e.g., policies related to the production and distribution of foods), to intermediate factors related to the characteristics of the living and working environments (e.g., access to healthy foods, physical activity resources), and to personal characteristics (e.g., genetic predisposition, behavioral choices). Health system factors also affect blood pressure levels through access to and quality of care. Additional examples of relevant factors at different levels are shown in Figure 1-3. This figure served as a heuristic to help the committee to think about the multiple factors that influence the population blood pressure distribution, the incidence and prevalence of hypertension, and blood pressure control; it was not intended to be a full representation of the many factors affecting blood pressure or to concretely specify the inter-relationships among the factors.

Within each of the levels shown in Figure 1-3, some factors may affect primarily the population distribution of blood pressure, whereas others may affect primarily the health consequences of hypertension (which in turn depend on early detection, treatment, and control of high blood pressure). In general the more "macro" factors (sometimes termed population-level factors) will affect primarily the distribution of blood pressure; in contrast the adequate control of high blood pressure will likely require the consid-

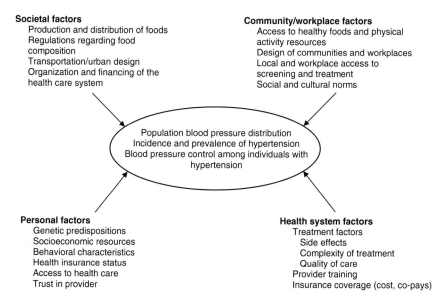

FIGURE 1-3 Schematic framework of factors affecting blood pressure.

eration of personal factors. However, these distinctions are not clear-cut. For example, societal factors related to the sodium content of processed foods may primarily affect the population distribution of blood pressure, but may also have important effects on blood pressure control among individuals diagnosed with hypertension. In addition, blood pressure control, including adherence to medication, among hypertensive individuals will be affected by personal factors such as health insurance status, access to providers, socioeconomic resources and other behavioral factors, but may also be impacted by societal health system organization as well as access to follow-up and monitoring in communities and workplaces.

In considering possible strategies for the prevention of high blood pressure and its adverse health consequences, the committee was guided by two basic features of the general framework illustrated in Figure 1-3: (1) the need to consider strategies aimed at shifting the population distribution of blood pressure (and thus preventing high blood pressure) as well as those targeted at persons considered to have hypertension based on current guidelines (to prevent the adverse consequences of high blood pressure); and (2) the need to consider factors at multiple levels, from societal to personal. Multiple categorizations of the possible interventions are possible. For simplicity, in this report, interventions are categorized in two broad domains: (1) population-wide strategies aimed at preventing high blood pressure by shifting the population distribution (referred to as population-based strategies) and (2) targeted strategies directed toward persons with, or at high risk, of high blood pressure aimed at reducing the adverse health consequences of hypertension through the early detection, treatment, and control hypertension (referred to as individual-based strategies).

Criteria for Identifying and Prioritizing Interventions

The committee developed a series of criteria to identify and prioritize recommended strategies and interventions. It was recognized that the information available to assess each of these criteria is highly variable and sometimes limited. Nevertheless it was agreed that public health decisions and recommendations need to be based on the best available evidence to date, with the recognition that the evidence may not be perfect and may evolve over time. No attempt was made to give specific weights to each of these criteria; rather they were used by the committee as general qualitative guidelines to help identify the most promising strategies for the CDC to pursue at this juncture. The criteria represent various domains relevant to prioritizing the CDC's strategy. Two criteria (potential impact on population prevalence and evidence of effectiveness) assess the expected impact of the intervention on hypertension at the population level. A third criterion (relative cost or feasibility) incorporates the practical issues of cost

TABLE 1-2 Criteria Considered for Selecting Priority Areas for the Prevention and Control of Hypertension

Criteria	Defining Questions	Considerations
Impact	To what extent will the strategy or intervention reduce the incidence of hypertension or complications associated with hypertension?	Effect size Proportion of people potentially affected
Effectiveness	What is the evidence of the strategy or intervention's impact in real-world settings?	Degree of generalizability to uncontrolled environments
Relative cost or feasibility	Is the strategy or intervention cost-effective? Qualitatively, how expensive is it to implement?	Cost-effectiveness analysis
Uniqueness	Is there a special role for the CDC and its partners in implementing the strategy or intervention?	Organizational authorities and mandates and roles
Synergy with other CDC programs	Will the strategy or intervention leverage or duplicate activities in other CDC units or activities conducted by other partners?	Division for Heart Disease and Stroke Prevention core efforts and resources
Reduction in disparities	Will the strategy or intervention reduce disparities in risk factors or health care?	Opportunity to narrow gaps in risk, disease burden, and care

and feasibility. Two additional criteria (unique contribution of the CDC and synergy among other CDC programs) consider specific issues related to the role of the CDC. Finally, the last criterion considers whether the interventions are likely to benefit the most vulnerable groups and reduce disparities. A brief description of each of the criteria is provided below and in Table 1-2.

Potential Impacts of Interventions on Population Prevalence of Hypertension (or distribution of blood pressure) and on Adverse Health Consequences

This first criterion assesses the potential impact of the intervention on the prevalence of hypertension (or its complications). Impact is a function of (1) the effect size of the intervention (as assessed by the relative risk or the risk difference) and (2) the proportion of people with the risk factor or condition at which the intervention is directed. Population impact is assessed through the calculation of the population attributable risk defined as the expected percentage reduction in the prevalence or incidence of the outcome in the population if the intervention were implemented in an ideal setting (i.e., the risk factor was entirely eliminated). The committee commissioned a review of the best available evidence on population attributable risk of a number of interventions intended to prevent hypertension. Although the ideal evidence would incorporate information on changes in blood pressure distributions rather than changes in arbitrarily defined dichotomous outcomes, very little information on the former exists. However, it is reasonable to make the assumption that the prevalence or incidence of hypertension is at least partly a function of the underlying blood pressure distribution.

The potential benefits of interventions focused on the early detection, treatment, and control of hypertension are also considered. In this case the potential benefit is not the prevention of hypertension but the reduction of its adverse health consequences through early detection, treatment, and control of individuals with hypertension (sometimes referred to as secondary prevention).

Evidence of Effectiveness in Real-World Settings

In addition to the potential impact of interventions (as quantified by the population attributable risk) based on effect sizes under ideal conditions (i.e., efficacy) and population prevalence, the committee also considered evidence of the impact or outcomes of interventions in practice or real-life settings. This real-life impact is sometimes referred to as effectiveness (Zaza et al., 2005). More generally, this criterion refers to the extent to which estimates of effect sizes of the intervention obtained from a given study (often conducted under ideal circumstances with excellent participation, fidelity of the intervention, and compliance) can be generalized to the slightly different circumstances that may arise in less controlled settings—for example, when the same intervention is implemented in the real world. Although efficacy and effectiveness are theoretically clearly distinguished in the extreme case, the extent to which a given study assesses efficacy or effectiveness is sometimes debatable. Therefore, the committee viewed this criterion in a qualitative way by considering the kinds of studies conducted and the extent to which their estimates are derived under conditions more akin to a laboratory or real-life setting.

Relative Cost or Feasibility

Despite the magnitude of hypertension-associated morbidity and mortality, current public health resources available for hypertension prevention and control are surprisingly limited, thus, hypertension interventions must be prioritized not only by effectiveness but also by cost, including both cost-effectiveness and absolute cost. Where possible, the committee reviewed available data on the cost of potential interventions and current DHDSP resources.

Unique Contribution of the CDC and Partner Agencies

In general, the CDC and state and local public health agencies are more experienced and skilled in population-based interventions than in interventions that provide health care directly to individuals. Government public health agencies are the only organizations with the mandate to provide population-wide services. Through leadership and convening strategies, government public health agencies can galvanize political commitment, develop policy, prioritize funding, and coordinate programs (Baker and Porter, 2005). In general, direct interventions providing health care to individuals (treatment) are much more distant from the unique skills and value-added of the CDC and state and local health partners.

Synergy with Other CDC Programs and Gap Analysis

Risk factors for and consequences of hypertension are common, overlap with other health conditions, and play a very large role in our overall population health. Thus, there already is substantial activity and prevention programming in place at the CDC and in state and local health departments. CDC priorities for hypertension prevention and control should not be duplicative of, but rather synergistic with, existing prevention programs in place within the CDC and in state and local health departments and in the community or individual health care settings. A similar dynamic of cross-cutting activities should, in theory, be present for health care interventions for communities or individuals.

Intervention Would Benefit the Most Vulnerable Groups
and Reduce Disparities in Hypertension

Hypertension is so common that broad-based interventions are essential. That said, it is also a disease for which there are major inequities across racial and economic groups—along the entire spectrum from risk factors to the delivery of medical care. Interventions directed toward general population groups historically do not correct these inequities and can even worsen them. Care was taken to identify a portfolio of interventions that might minimize existing inequities in the prevention, detection, and control of hypertension.

Hypertension is also a disease of aging, becoming increasingly prevalent as one grows older. From the perspective of the proportion affected, attention must be directed toward groups with the highest prevalence. However, from the perspective of the individual, hypertension in younger age groups has a greater potential for causing premature morbidity and mortality, so special attention needs to be paid to this at-risk population.

In the next chapters the committee reviews trends in hypertension and then applies the framework and criteria, to the extent possible, to the selection of priority strategies for the CDC and its partners.

REFERENCES

Ahern, J., M. R. Jones, E. Bakshis, and S. Galea. 2008. Revisiting Rose: Comparing the benefits and costs of population-wide and targeted interventions. *Milbank Quarterly* 86(4):581-600.

AHRQ (Agency for Healthcare Research and Quality). 2007. *Screening for high blood pressure.* Rockville, MD: U.S. Preventive Services Task Force.

ALLHAT (Antihypertensive and Lipid-Lowering Treatment to Prevent Heart Attack Trial). 2002. Major outcomes in high-risk hypertensive patients randomized to angiotensin-converting enzyme inhibitor or calcium channel blocker vs diuretic: The Antihypertensive and Lipid-Lowering Treatment to Prevent Heart Attack Trial (ALLHAT). *Journal of the American Medical Association* 288(23):2981-2997.

Baker, E. L., and J. Porter. 2005. Practicing management and leadership: Creating the information network for public health officials. *Journal of Public Health Management and Practice* 11(5):469-473.

Balu, S., and J. Thomas, 3rd. 2006. Incremental expenditure of treating hypertension in the United States. *American Journal of Hypertension* 19(8):810-816.

CDC (Centers for Disease Control and Prevention). 2006. *Healthy People 2010 Midcourse Review: Section 12: Heart disease and stroke.* http://www.healthypeople.gov/data/mid course/pdf/fa12.pdf (accessed February 4, 2010).

Chobanian, A. V., G. L. Bakris, H. R. Black, W. C. Cushman, L. A. Green, J. L. Izzo, Jr., D. W. Jones, B. J. Materson, S. Oparil, J. T. Wright, Jr., and E. J. Roccella. 2003. The Seventh Report of the Joint National Committee on Prevention, Detection, Evaluation, and Treatment of High Blood Pressure: The JNC 7 Report. *Journal of the American Medical Association* 289(19):2560-2572.

Cutler, D. M., G. Long, E. R. Berndt, J. Royer, A. A. Fournier, A. Sasser, and P. Cremieux. 2007. The value of antihypertensive drugs: A perspective on medical innovation. *Health Affairs* 26(1):97-110.

Danaei, G., E. L. Ding, D. Mozaffarian, B. Taylor, J. Rehm, C. J. Murray, and M. Ezzati. 2009. The preventable causes of death in the United States: Comparative risk assessment of dietary, lifestyle, and metabolic risk factors. *PLoS Medicine* 6(4):e1000058.

DeVol, R., and A. Bedroussian. 2007. *An unhealthy America: The economic burden of chronic disease.* Santa Monica, CA: Milken Institute.

Fields, L. E., V. L. Burt, J. A. Cutler, J. Hughes, E. J. Roccella, and P. Sorlie. 2004. The burden of adult hypertension in the United States 1999 to 2000: A rising tide. *Hypertension* 44(4):398-404.

Lloyd-Jones, D., R. Adams, M. Carnethon, G. De Simone, T. B. Ferguson, K. Flegal, E. Ford, K. Furie, A. Go, K. Greenlund, N. Haase, S. Hailpern, M. Ho, V. Howard, B. Kissela, S. Kittner, D. Lackland, L. Lisabeth, A. Marelli, M. McDermott, J. Meigs, D. Mozaffarian, G. Nichol, C. O'Donnell, V. Roger, W. Rosamond, R. Sacco, P. Sorlie, R. Stafford, J. Steinberger, T. Thom, S. Wasserthiel-Smoller, N. Wong, J. Wylie-Rosett, and Y. Hong. 2009. Heart disease and stroke statistics—2009 update: A report from the American Heart Association Statistics Committee and Stroke Statistics Subcommittee. *Circulation* 119(3):480-486.

Miller, G. E., and M. Zodet. 2006. *Trends in the pharmaceutical treatment of hypertension, 1997 to 2003. Research findings no. 25.* http://meps.ahrq.gov/mepsweb/data_files/publications/rf25/rf25.pdf (accessed January 20, 1010).

NHLBI (National Heart, Lung, and Blood Institute). 2004a. *JNC7 media kit.* http://www.nhlbi.nih.gov/guidelines/hypertension/media_kit.htm (accessed January 27, 2010).

———. 2004b. *Prevent and control America's high blood pressure: Mission possible.* Bethesda, MD: National Institutes of Health.

Psaty, B. M., T. A. Manolio, N. L. Smith, S. R. Heckbert, J. S. Gottdiener, G. L. Burke, J. Weissfeld, P. Enright, T. Lumley, N. Powe, and C. D. Furberg. 2002. Time trends in high blood pressure control and the use of antihypertensive medications in older adults: The Cardiovascular Health Study. *Archives of Internal Medicine* 162(20):2325-2332.

Rose, G. 2001. Sick individuals and sick populations. *International Journal of Epidemiology* 30(3):427-432.

Vasan, R. S., A. Beiser, S. Seshadri, M. G. Larson, W. B. Kannel, R. B. D'Agostino, and D. Levy. 2002. Residual lifetime risk for developing hypertension in middle-aged women and men: The Framingham Heart Study. *Journal of the American Medical Association* 287(8):1003-1010.

Whelton, P. K., J. He, L. J. Appel, J. A. Cutler, S. Havas, T. A. Kotchen, E. J. Roccella, R. Stout, C. Vallbona, M. C. Winston, and J. Karimbakas. 2002. Primary prevention of hypertension: Clinical and public health advisory from the National High Blood Pressure Education Program. *Journal of the American Medical Association* 288(15):1882-1888.

Zaza, S., P. A. Briss, and K. Harris (editors). 2005. *The guide to community preventive services: What works to promote health?* Task Force on Community Preventive Services. London, UK: Oxford University Press.

2

Public Health Importance of Hypertension

Hypertension is an important public health challenge in the United States and other countries due to its high prevalence and strong association with cardiovascular disease and premature death (Cutler et al., 2008; Fields et al., 2004; Gu et al., 2002; Kearney et al., 2005; Lawes et al., 2008). Approximately 73 million U.S. adults (35 million men and 38 million women) had hypertension in 2006 (Lloyd-Jones et al., 2009). The estimated total number of adults with hypertension in the world in 2000 was 972 million: 333 million in economically developed countries and 639 million in economically developing countries (Kearney et al., 2005).

Hypertension is not only the most common, but also one of the most important, modifiable risk factors for coronary heart disease, stroke, congestive heart failure, chronic kidney disease, and peripheral vascular disease (Collins et al., 1990; Gu et al., 2008; Hebert et al., 1993; Kannel, 1996; Klag et al., 1996; Lewington et al., 2002; MacMahon et al., 1990; Staessen et al., 2001; Stamler et al., 1993; Whelton, 1994). The positive relationship between blood pressure and the risk of vascular disease is strong, continuous, graded, consistent, independent, predictive, and etiologically significant for those with and without a previous history of cardiovascular disease (He et al., 2003). Systolic blood pressure is a more important risk factor for cardiovascular disease than diastolic blood pressure (Gu et al., 2008; Klag et al., 1996; Stamler et al., 1993). Hypertension has also been identified as one of the leading preventable risk factors for all-cause mortality and is ranked third as a cause of disability-adjusted life-years (Ezzati et al., 2002; Lawes et al., 2008). Furthermore, randomized controlled trials have demonstrated that antihypertensive drug treatment reduces vascular disease incidence and mortality among patients with hypertension (Collins et al., 1990; Ezzati et al., 2002; Hebert et al., 1993; Staessen et al., 2001).

PREVALENCE OF HYPERTENSION IN THE U.S. POPULATION

This section provides a discussion of the burden of hypertension by age, gender, and race or ethnicity and reviews data on levels of awareness, treatment, and control of hypertension. The relationship between behavioral risk factors and hypertension is addressed in Chapter 4, but trends in select risk factors are provided here.

The prevalence of hypertension in the U.S. general population is high and increasing in recent years (Cutler et al., 2008; Fields et al., 2004). The National Health and Nutrition Examination Survey (NHANES) conducted by the National Center for Health Statistics has been the principal means of tracking the burden of hypertension in the U.S. general population. Hypertension prevalence estimates derived from the NHANES are defined as systolic blood pressure ≥140 mm Hg and/or diastolic blood pressure ≥90 mm Hg and/or receiving antihypertensive medication.

The estimated prevalence of hypertension derived from the NHANES 1999-2004 was 28.9 percent of the U.S. adult population (Cutler et al., 2008). The prevalence of hypertension varies by age, gender, and race or ethnicity. The prevalence of hypertension is also affected by behavior such as the intake of dietary sodium and potassium, weight management, alcohol consumption, and physical activity. Overall, the prevalence of hypertension is similar in men and women in the United States. In the NHANES 1999-2004, the age-adjusted prevalence of hypertension for all races was 28.5 percent in men and 28.8 percent in women (Cutler et al., 2008). The relationship between gender and hypertension is modified by age. In young adults, the prevalence of hypertension is higher in men than in women. However, by their fifties, women tend to have blood pressure levels that equal or exceed those of men. The prevalence of hypertension is higher in women than in men later in life. The increase in the prevalence of hypertension by race and sex between the age groups of 18-29 years of age and >70 years of age was from 9.8 to 83.4 percent in black men, from 3.7 to 83.1 percent in black women, from 3.5 to 69.1 percent in Mexican-American men, from 1.5 to 78.8 percent in Mexican-American women, from 5.5 to 63.3 percent in non-Hispanic white men, and from 0.8 to 78.8 in non-Hispanic white women (Table 2-1). Isolated systolic hypertension (defined as systolic blood pressure ≥140 mm Hg and diastolic blood pressure <90 mm Hg) is common in older persons because systolic blood pressure tends to rise until the eighth or ninth decade, whereas diastolic blood pressure tends to remain constant or decline after the fifth decade (Whelton, 1994).

TABLE 2-1 Age-Specific Prevalence (Standard Error) of Hypertension in the U.S. Adult Population: NHANES 1999-2004

Age (years)	Non-Hispanic White		Non-Hispanic Black		Mexican American	
	Men	Women	Men	Women	Men	Women
18-29	5.5 (1.1)	0.8 (0.3)	9.8 (1.9)	3.7 (1.0)	3.5 (1.1)	1.5 (0.6)
30-39	12.5 (1.9)	5.4 (1.0)	18.5 (2.5)	14.5 (2.9)	10.6 (2.7)	5.7 (1.8)
40-49	23.9 (2.1)	19.9 (2.1)	33.6 (2.8)	45.0 (3.0)	23.7 (2.4)	20.5 (3.0)
50-59	36.5 (3.0)	39.8 (2.7)	57.3 (4.1)	61.2 (4.3)	30.4 (4.2)	38.9 (4.8)
60-69	56.0 (2.3)	58.4 (2.2)	74.2 (2.8)	84.1 (2.6)	53.2 (3.4)	62.7 (2.6)
≥70	63.3 (1.7)	78.8 (1.5)	83.4 (3.3)	83.1 (3.5)	69.1 (3.5)	78.8 (3.3)
Total	27.5 (1.1)	26.9 (0.7)	39.1 (1.1)	40.8 (1.2)	26.2 (1.2)	27.5 (1.3)

SOURCE: Adapted from Cutler et al., 2008.

The age-adjusted prevalence of hypertension among those surveyed in the NHANES 1999-2004 was highest among non-Hispanic blacks at 40.1 percent, compared to 27.4 percent in non-Hispanic whites and 27.1 percent in Mexican Americans. Non-Hispanic blacks also had the highest prevalence of hypertension among all races or ethnicities for every age group and for both gender groups (Cutler et al., 2008).

Hypertension in Children and Adolescents

The prevalence of high blood pressure among children and adolescents has been examined in the NHANES and other studies (Berenson et al., 2006; Din-Dzietham et al., 2007; Ostchega et al., 2009). Based on guidelines detailed in the *Fourth Report on the Diagnosis, Evaluation, and Treatment of High Blood Pressure in Children and Adolescents*, high blood pressure is defined as having systolic and/or diastolic blood pressure that ranks as ≥95th percentile for gender, age, and height (National High Blood Pressure Education Program Working Group on High Blood Pressure in Children and Adolescents, 2004). The guidelines recommend multiple blood pressure measurements at different times to define persistent high blood pressure. However, blood pressure was measured at only one clinic visit for the NHANES and thus might overestimate prevalence. Overall, the prevalence of elevated blood pressure during the period 2003 to 2006 was 2.6 percent in boys and 3.4 percent in girls ages 8-17 years in the United States (Ostchega et al., 2009). The gender- and race- or ethnicity-specific prevalence was 2.5 percent and 3.8 percent in non-Hispanic white boys and girls; among non-Hispanic black boys and girls it was 2.8 percent and 3.7 percent respectively, and among Mexican-American boys and girls it was 2.4 percent and 1.7 percent, respectively (Table 2-2).

Secular Trends in the Prevalence of Hypertension

Effective monitoring and surveillance systems need to be in place to monitor progress in reducing the prevalence of hypertension and increasing the awareness, treatment, and control of hypertension. Repeated independent cross-sectional surveys in the same populations over time can provide important information about secular trends in blood pressure. However, attention must be paid to the comparability of survey methods with respect to sampling and blood pressure measurement as well as the definition of hypertension. In the general U.S. population, government surveys (NHES I [National Health Examination Survey]; NHANES I, II, and III; HHANES [Hispanic Health and Nutrition Examination Survey]) may provide the best data to examine secular trends in hypertension; however, there have been significant modifications in the protocol for blood pressure measurement,

TABLE 2-2 Prevalence (Standard Error) of Elevated Blood Pressure[a] Among Children and Adolescents Ages 8 Through 17 Years: NHANES 2003-2006

Age (years)	Non-Hispanic White		Non-Hispanic Black		Mexican American	
	Boys	Girls	Boys	Girls	Boys	Girls
8-12	3.6 (1.2)	3.9 (1.2)	2.7 (1.2)	4.2 (1.4)	2.1 (1.0)	1.9 (0.8)
13-17	1.6 (0.7)	3.7 (1.3)	2.9 (0.7)	3.1 (0.8)	2.7 (0.8)	1.5 (0.6)
Total	2.5 (0.7)	3.8 (1.0)	2.8 (0.6)	3.7 (0.9)	2.4 (0.6)	1.7 (0.5)

[a] Elevated blood pressure was defined as average systolic blood pressure and/or diastolic blood pressure that is ≥95th percentile for gender, age, and height.
SOURCE: Adapted from Ostchega et al., 2009.

sample sizes, and other factors that make these data not completely comparable (Burt et al., 1995).

Between 1960 and the early 1990s, blood pressure data collection changed in significant ways. Changes include the number of measurements taken per occasion (one, two, or three measures before 1988; two sets of three measures after 1988); the number of occasions that blood pressure was measured (one or two occasions); and the posture in which blood pressure was taken (sitting or supine). Current national guidelines recommend three blood pressure measurements on multiple days for a clinical diagnosis of hypertension. One blood pressure measurement taken on a single occasion cannot represent the usual blood pressure level of individuals because of random variation in the measurement over time. The first blood pressure measurement, for example, is typically higher than subsequent measurements. Further, blood pressure can also be subject to the white coat effect[1] (Chobanian et al., 2003; Pickering et al., 2005).

Another important change is the size of blood pressure cuffs available to measure blood pressure. In early years (1960-1962), adult blood pressure cuffs were primarily used; over time, blood pressure cuffs suitable for children and different adult size cuffs were added (adult large and thigh cuff). Blood pressure measurements could be biased if the cuff size is too small or too large relative to the patient's arm circumference (Pickering et al., 2005). There were also differences in maintenance of the blood pressure equipment used (unknown, daily, weekly, monthly calibration protocols). The personnel responsible for taking blood pressures varied (physician, nurse, or interviewer) as did the levels of training received (unknown, 1.5 days or 3 days).

The quality of blood pressure measurements is partially reflected by the digit preference. A high proportion of zero-end digits in blood pressure measures indicated the poor quality of blood pressure measurement. Approximately one-half of blood pressure measures had a zero-end digit in the NHANES 1971-1974 and 1976-1980 compared to approximately one-quarter in the NHANES 1988-1991 (Burt et al., 1995). In addition, the definition of diastolic blood pressure changed from measurement at the fourth Korotkoff sound (muffling of sound and point of disappearance) to the fifth Korotkoff sound (complete cessation of sound, NHANES III). Finally, the definitions used to define hypertension changed from 160/95 mm Hg in earlier studies to 140/90 mm Hg in the NHANES III (Chobanian et al., 2003). This change, in particular, has made it more difficult to determine secular trends. Having noted these methodological issues, the next

---

[1] A white coat effect refers to higher blood pressure readings when taken by a health care provider or in a medical setting than would occur if blood pressure were taken at home.

section describes the secular trends in hypertension based upon available data.

Based on the NHANES surveys, the prevalence of hypertension in the U.S. adult population generally declined between 1971 and 1991 (Burt et al., 1995). The decline in the prevalence of hypertension was consistent across age, gender, and racial groups. For example, the age-adjusted prevalence of hypertension defined as blood pressure ≥140/90 mm Hg and/or current use of antihypertensive medication decreased from 48.2 percent in blacks (49.0 percent in men and 47.5 percent in women) in 1971-1974 to 30.2 percent in blacks (32.6 percent in men and 28.1 percent in women) in 1988-1991. A similar decrease was seen among whites; hypertension prevalence decreased from 35.0 percent in 1971-1974 (40.1 percent in men and 30.2 percent in women) to 19.2 percent (21.6 percent in men and 16.7 percent in women) in 1988-1991 (Burt et al., 1995). However, the prevalence of hypertension began to increase in the later NHANES surveys. For example, the age-standardized prevalence among U.S. adults ages 18 years and older increased from 24.4 to 28.9 percent (p < 0.001) between the NHANES 1988-1994 and the NHANES 1999-2004, with the largest increases among non-Hispanic women from 21.7 to 26.9 (Cutler et al., 2008). The change in hypertension prevalence seems independent from the obesity epidemic in the U.S. population because the secular trends of hypertension were consistent across body mass index categories (<25.0, 25.0-29.9, and ≥30.0 kg/m^2) (Gregg et al., 2005).

Secular Trends Among the Elderly

Ostchega and colleagues reported a significant increase in hypertension prevalence in the U.S. population among those ages 60 years and older from 1988 to 2004. The prevalence of hypertension in the total population increased from 58 percent in the NHANES 1988-1994 to 67 percent in the NHANES 1999-2004 (Ostchega et al., 2007). A significant increase was seen in each age group studied (60-69: from 48 to 60 percent; 70-79: from 62 to 72 percent; and ≥80: from 69 to 77 percent), in both sexes (men: from 54 to 61 percent; women: from 60 to 72 percent). Figure 2-1 shows the increase in hypertension prevalence by age group and gender (Ostchega et al., 2007). Hypertension prevalence also increased in three racial or ethnicity categories (non-Hispanic whites: from 56 to 66 percent; non-Hispanic blacks: from 71 to 82 percent; and Mexican American: 62 to 68 percent).

Secular Trends in Children

Secular trends in mean blood pressure level and hypertension prevalence among children and adolescents ages 8 to 17 years were examined

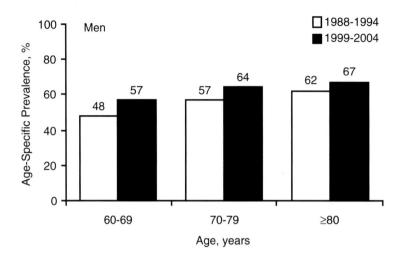

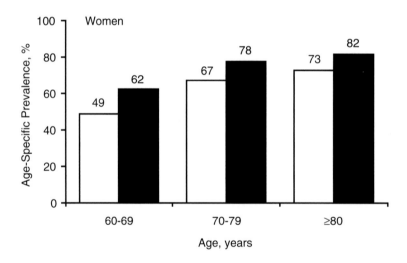

FIGURE 2-1 Age-specific prevalence of hypertension in U.S. adults ages 60 and older for men and women, NHANES 1988-1994 and NHANES 1999-2004. SOURCE: Adapted from Ostchega et al., 2007.

by various investigators using data from the NHANES (Din-Dzietham et al., 2007; Ostchega et al., 2007, 2009). Muntner and colleagues found that mean systolic blood pressure increased between 1988-1994 and 1999-2000. After controlling for differences in age, race, and sex, they found a 1.4 mm Hg increase in systolic blood pressure and a 3.3 mm Hg increase in diastolic blood pressure between the two surveys. The greatest differences were increases in mean systolic blood pressure (2.3 mm Hg increase) and mean diastolic blood pressure (4.4 mm Hg increase) of Mexican-American children. The increase in mean systolic and diastolic blood pressure was also higher in children ages 8 to 12 years compared to children ages 13-17 years (Muntner et al., 2004).

A more recent analysis of NHANES data surveys conducted in 1988-1994, 1999-2002, and 2003-2006 also shows an overall increase in elevated blood pressure in children and adolescents ages 8 though 17 years (Ostchega et al., 2009). The percent prevalence of elevated blood pressure

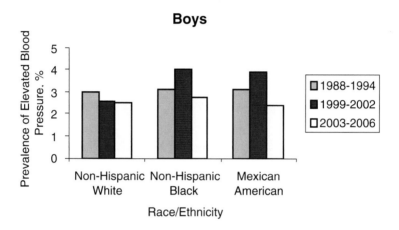

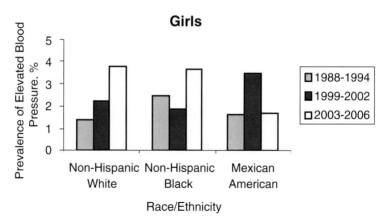

FIGURE 2-2 Prevalence of elevated blood pressure among children and adolescents ages 8 through 17 years: United States, NHANES 1988-1994, 1999-2002, and 2003-2006.
SOURCE: Adapted from Ostchega et al., 2009.

increased from 2.1 percent in 1988-1994 to 3.0 percent in 2003-2006. In the 2003-2006 survey, 2.6 percent of boys and 3.4 percent of girls had elevated blood pressure. Figure 2-2 shows the prevalence of elevated blood pressure by gender and race or ethnicity. After conducting multivariate analyses controlling for weight status, age, and race and ethnicity, the authors concluded that the prevalence of elevated blood pressure increased among girls ages 8-17 but had decreased among boys ages 13-17.

Incidence and Lifetime Risk of Hypertension

Although the prevalence of hypertension is a useful indicator of the burden of disease in the community, it does not provide information regarding the risk for individuals of developing hypertension. The individual risk for developing hypertension is best described by incidence or lifetime cumulative incidence statistics. Limited information is available about the incidence of hypertension because it requires follow-up of a large population for a prolonged period of time (Apostolides et al., 1982; Cornoni-Huntley et al., 1989; Fuchs et al., 2001; Manolio et al., 1994).

Several longitudinal cohort studies have shown that African Americans have a higher incidence of hypertension than whites (Apostolides et al., 1982; Cornoni-Huntley et al., 1989; Fuchs et al., 2001; Manolio et al., 1994). In the Atherosclerosis Risk in Communities Study, the 6-year incidence of hypertension was 13.9 percent and 12.6 percent in white men and women, and 24.9 percent and 30.3 percent in African-American men and women, ages 45-49 years, respectively (Fuchs et al., 2001). The corresponding incidence of hypertension among participants ages 50-64 years was 18.0 percent and 17.0 percent in white men and women, and 28.3 percent and 29.9 percent in African-American men and women, respectively. Other longitudinal cohort studies indicated that the incidence of hypertension in African Americans was an average of two times higher than in whites (Apostolides et al., 1982; Cornoni-Huntley et al., 1989; Manolio et al., 1994).

The lifetime risk for developing hypertension was estimated among 1,298 study participants who were 55 to 65 years of age and free of hypertension at baseline during 1976-1998 (Vasan et al., 2002). For 55-year-old participants, the cumulative risk of developing hypertension was calculated through age 80, while for 65-year-old participants, the risk for developing hypertension was calculated through age 85. These follow-up time intervals (25 years for 55-year-olds and 20 years for 65-year-olds) correspond to the current average number of remaining years of life for white individuals at these two ages in the United States. The lifetime risk for developing hypertension was 90 percent for both 55- and 65-year-old participants

(Figure 2-3). The lifetime probability of receiving antihypertensive medication was 60 percent (Vasan et al., 2002).

INTERNATIONAL COMPARISON

Kearney and colleagues estimated the global burden of hypertension in 2000 by pooling prevalence data from different regions of the world (Kearney et al., 2005). In their estimation, overall, 26.4 percent of the worldwide adult population ages 20 years and older in 2000 had hypertension (26.6 percent of men and 26.1 percent of women). The prevalence of hypertension varied greatly by world regions. For men, the highest estimated prevalence was in Latin America and the Caribbean (40.7 percent), and for women, the highest estimated prevalence was in the former socialist economies (39.1 percent). The lowest estimated prevalence of hypertension for both men (17.0 percent) and women (14.5 percent) was in the region encompassing Asia and the Pacific Islands. In comparison, the prevalence of hypertension in the U.S. adult population was 28.9 percent (NHANES 1999-2004), slightly higher than the estimated world prevalence of 26.4 percent (Cutler et al., 2008).

Hypertension is costly to the global health care system. A recent analysis by Gaziano et al. (2009), estimated that the global direct medical cost of nonoptimal blood pressure (defined as systolic blood pressure above 115 mm Hg and includes prehypertension and hypertension) was US $370 billion for the year 2001. This cost represents about 10 percent of global healthcare expenditures (Gaziano et al., 2009).

AWARENESS, TREATMENT, AND CONTROL OF HYPERTENSION IN THE COMMUNITY

Treatment and control of hypertension in the community requires that elevated blood pressure be recognized and that individuals with hypertension receive adequate treatment. In the United States, there has been remarkable improvement in the awareness, treatment, and control of hypertension since the late 1970s (Burt et al., 1995; Cutler et al., 2008; Hajjar and Kotchen, 2003; Ostchega et al., 2007). The proportion of hypertensive patients who are aware of their condition increased from 51 percent (42 percent in men and 63 percent in women) in the NHANES 1976-1980 to 69 percent (62 percent in men and 75 percent in women) in the NHANES 1988-1994 to 72 percent (69 percent in men and 74 percent in women) in the NHANES 1999-2004 (Burt et al., 1995; Cutler et al., 2008). The increase in awareness of hypertension between 1976-1980 and 1999-2004 was accompanied by an increase in the proportion of individuals with hypertension who receive treatment with antihypertensive medications. Over-

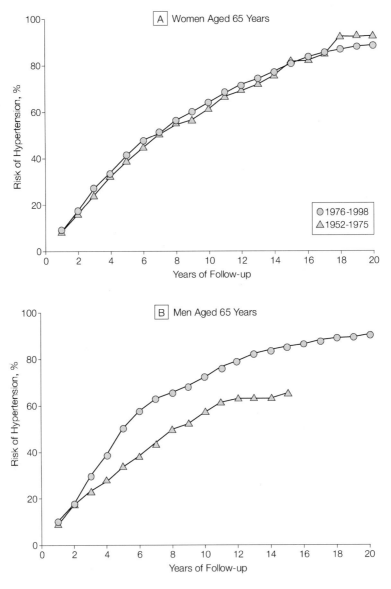

FIGURE 2-3 Residual lifetime risk of hypertension in women and men aged 65 years. Cumulative incidence of hypertension in 65-year-old women and men. Data for 65-year-old men in the 1952-1975 period are truncated at 15 years since there were few participants in this age category who were followed up beyond this time. SOURCE: Vasan et al., *Journal of the American Medical Association*, February 27, 2002, 287:1008. Copyright © (2002) American Medical Association. All rights reserved.

all, the percentage of individuals with hypertension who receive treatment increased from 31 percent (21 percent in men and 43 percent in women) in the NHANES 1976-1980 to 53 percent (45 percent in men and 61 percent in women) in the NHANES 1988-1994 to 61 percent (58 percent in men and 65 percent in women) in the NHANES 1999-2004. The proportion of controlled hypertension increased more than threefold at the 140/90 mm Hg cut-point from 10 percent (5 percent in men and 15 percent in women) in the NHANES 1976-1980 to 26 percent (21 percent in men and 31 percent in women) in the NHANES 1988-1994 to 35 percent (36 percent in men and 34 percent in women) in the NHANES 1999-2004 (Burt et al., 1995; Cutler et al., 2008).

The degree of awareness, treatment, and control (blood pressure <140/90 mm Hg) of hypertension varies considerably by gender, race or ethnicity, socioeconomic status, education, and quality of health care (He et al., 2002; Hyman and Pavlik, 2001; Muntner et al., 2004). Differences in gender and race or ethnicity are considered here. Based on the NHANES 1999-2004 data, black women have the highest awareness (81.8 percent) and treatment (71.7 percent) rates, while white men have the highest control (39.3 percent) rate (Table 2-3). On the other hand, Mexican-American men have the lowest awareness (55.9 percent), treatment (40.4 percent), and control (21.4 percent) rates. Awareness and treatment rates were higher for women than men across all racial or ethnic groups. The control rate was higher for women among blacks and Mexican Americans but higher for men among whites (Cutler et al., 2008).

Among individuals with untreated or uncontrolled hypertension, elevated systolic blood pressure with a diastolic pressure of less than 90 mm Hg often remains a problem. Hyman and Pavlik, using the same NHANES data set, conducted an analysis of blood pressure levels in individuals with uncontrolled hypertension (Hyman and Pavlik, 2001). They found that close to 80 percent of individuals with hypertension present but who were unaware had a systolic blood pressure ≥140 mm Hg and a diastolic blood pressure <90 mm Hg.

The actual awareness, treatment, and control rates are likely higher than the NHANES estimates due to the definition of hypertension in the study. In the NHANES, the diagnosis of hypertension was based on blood pressure measurement at a single clinical visit, whereas national guidelines recommend that the classification of hypertension be based on the mean of two or more blood pressure readings taken during two or more office visits (Chobanian et al., 2003). Thus, some of the individuals classified as unaware and untreated hypertensive might not meet the criteria for hypertension in the clinical setting.

Although the proportion of individuals with controlled hypertension has increased substantially, the majority (65 percent) of individuals with

TABLE 2-3 Hypertension Awareness, Treatment, and Control in the U.S. Adult Hypertensive Population: NHANES 1988-1994 and NHANES 1999-2004

	Awareness (%)		Treatment (%)		Control (%)	
	1988-1994	1999-2004	1988-1994	1999-2004	1988-1994	1999-2004
Total	68.5	71.8	53.1	61.4	26.1	35.1
Men	61.6	69.3	44.6	57.9	20.7	36.2
Women	74.8	73.9	61.0	64.5	31.2	34.2
Non-Hispanic white	69.1	72.0	54.2	62.1	27.3	36.8
Men	63.0	70.4	46.2	60.0	22.0	39.3
Women	74.7	73.4	61.6	64.0	32.2	34.5
Non-Hispanic black	71.0	75.8	54.8	65.1	24.0	33.4
Men	62.5	67.8	42.3	56.4	16.6	29.9
Women	77.8	81.8	64.6	71.7	30.0	36.0
Mexican American	57.5	61.3	38.6	47.4	16.2	24.3
Men	47.8	55.9	30.9	40.4	13.5	21.4
Women	69.3	66.9	47.8	54.9	19.4	27.4

SOURCE: Adapted from Cutler et al., 2008.

hypertension are not under control. Wang and Vasan (2005) highlighted factors associated with uncontrolled hypertension in the United States, categorized by patient and physician factors. Patient factors related to uncontrolled hypertension include lack of insurance and provider, increased susceptibility due to advanced age and obesity, therapy nonadherence because of medication cost, complicated regimens, lack of social support, and poor physician-patient communication. Physician factors related to uncontrolled hypertension include lack of knowledge about guidelines, overestimating guideline adherence, concerns about medication side effects, and limited office visit time.

Many barriers to hypertension control in the general population affect African Americans, especially African-American men, disproportionally (Cooper, 2009). Barriers to hypertension include higher pre-treatment blood pressure levels, health care access and medication costs, social barriers related to urban life, personal barriers (i.e., tobacco, drug, and alcohol addiction), physician inertia in initiation and intensification of blood pressure medication, and time constraints during outpatient visits that impair physician-patient communication and patient adherence.

In general, compared to the United States, the rates of awareness, treatment, and control of hypertension were lower in other developed countries (Falaschetti et al., 2009; Joffres et al., 1997). The most recent Canadian Heart Health Surveys 1986-1992 for which data are available reported that 58 percent (53 percent in men and 65 percent in women) of individuals with hypertension were aware of their condition, 39 percent (32 percent in men and 49 percent in women) were treated, and 16 percent (13 percent in men and 20 percent in women) had their blood pressure controlled (Joffres et al., 1997). The Health Survey for England 2006 reported that the awareness, treatment, and control rates of hypertension were 66 percent (62 percent in men and 71 percent in women), 54 percent (47 percent in men and 62 percent in women), and 28 percent (24 percent in men and 32 percent in women), respectively (Falaschetti et al., 2009). The rates of awareness, treatment, and control of hypertension were even lower in developing countries. The China National Nutrition and Health Survey 2002 reported that among individuals with hypertension, only 24 percent were aware of their condition, 19 percent were receiving antihypertensive medications, and less than 5 percent had adequate control of blood pressure (Wu et al., 2008).

HYPERTENSION DATA QUALITY AND MONITORING CONCERNS

Throughout its review, the committee struggled to clearly understand the trends in hypertension over time. As noted earlier, government surveys (NHES I; NHANES I, II, and III; HHANES) that collect blood pressure data and related information (hypertension awareness) have varied significantly in their methods over the years. While methodological adjustments to reduce bias in survey data collected over 1971-1991 have allowed survey data to be compared, the degree to which these adjustments allow an accurate assessment of secular hypertension trends remains unclear especially since it is difficult to explain the pronounced reduction in hypertension prevalence over that period.

Therefore, at the request of the committee, the Centers for Disease Control and Prevention (CDC) provided unpublished data of secular trends in mean and median systolic and diastolic blood pressure and hypertension prevalence among children (8-17 years) and adults (20 years and above) based on the first blood pressure measurement taken from the National Health and Nutrition Examination Surveys from 1971 onward (NHANES I, 1971-1975; NHANES II, 1976-1980; NHANES III, 1988-1994; NHANES 1999-2002; NHANES 2003-2006). The data were provided in this way to minimize the problem of inconsistent number of blood pressure measurements taken over the survey periods and to facilitate comparison of the data over time (Table 2-4). The reader should note that even with this adjustment, data are insufficient to assess whether blood pressure levels and hypertension prevalence truly fell between 1971 and 1988, because other significant quality control problems with the 1971 survey are not accounted for in this analysis.

A comparison was made of the first blood pressure reading in the NHANES participants over time. The age-, sex-, and race-adjusted prevalence of hypertension in the U.S. adult population ages 20 years and older decreased from 41.1 percent in 1971-1975 to 28.6 in 2003-2006. The mean blood pressure also decreased from the early 1970s (systolic 131.5 and 138.6 mm Hg, and diastolic 82.5 and 87.4 mm Hg in whites and blacks, respectively) to the late of 1980s (systolic 121.7 and 127.5 mm Hg, and diastolic 73.0 and 75.5 mm Hg in whites and blacks, respectively) (Figure 2-4). This is partially due to differences in the definition of diastolic blood pressure (Korotkoff phase 4 or 5 in the NHANES 1971-1975 and Korotkoff phase 5 only in the NHANES 1988-1994) (Din-Dzietham et al., 2007). Subsequently, mean systolic blood pressure increased slightly and diastolic blood pressure decreased slightly during the 1990s and 2000s. These changes in mean blood pressure could reflect both changes in risk factors of blood pressure and treatment of hypertension.

A comparison of the first blood pressure measurement among children and adolescents ages 8-17 years from the NHANES over the same survey periods also found a significant decrease in hypertension. Hypertension prevalence dropped from 17.3 in 1971-1975 to 5.1 in 2003-2006.

Comparisons of the age- and sex-adjusted mean blood pressures during 1971-2006 (Figure 2-5) in children are also informative. The age- and sex-adjusted systolic blood pressure decreased from 110.1 mm Hg in

TABLE 2-4 Median and Mean Systolic and Diastolic Blood Pressure and Prevalence of Hypertension for Adults and Children Based on First Blood Pressure Measurement—NHANES Data

	1971-1975	1976-1980	1988-1994	1999-2002	2003-2006
Adults (20+)					
HTN prevalence (%) (SE)	41.1 (1.2)	42.0 (1.8)	21.2 (0.7)	27.0 (1.4)	28.6 (0.8)
Median systolic (mm Hg) (SE)	126.4 (1.1)	122.9 (1.5)	117.5 (0.3)	119.8 (0.5)	119.7 (0.3)
Mean systolic (mm Hg) (SE)	132.2 (0.4)	129.0 (0.6)	122.4 (0.3)	124.1 (0.4)	122.9 (0.4)
Median diastolic (mm Hg) (SE)	79.8 (0.1)	79.1 (0.2)	71.7 (0.3)	71.9 (0.3)	70.2 (0.3)
Mean diastolic (mm Hg) (SE)	82.0 (0.3)	81.3 (0.5)	73.4 (0.3)	72.7 (0.3)	70.9 (0.2)
Children (8-17 years)					
HTN prevalence (%) (SE)	17.3 (1.1)	15.8 (1.1)	3.8 (1.1)	4.9 (1.1)	5.1 (1.1)
Median systolic (mm Hg) (SE)	109.3 (0.1)	109.2 (0.5)	103.9 (0.5)	105.0 (0.4)	106.1 (0.4)
Mean systolic (mm Hg) (SE)	109.9 (0.5)	108.7 (0.6)	105.2 (0.4)	106.5 (0.2)	107.4 (0.4)
Median diastolic (mm Hg) (SE)	69.1 (.06)	69.3 (0.1)	57.0 (0.5)	59.5 (0.04)	56.2 (0.5)
Mean diastolic (mm Hg) (SE)	68.1 (0.4)	69.0 (0.4)	57.2 (0.4)	60.2 (0.4)	56.8 (0.4)

NOTE: HTN = hypertension; SE = standard error.
SOURCE: CDC unpublished data.

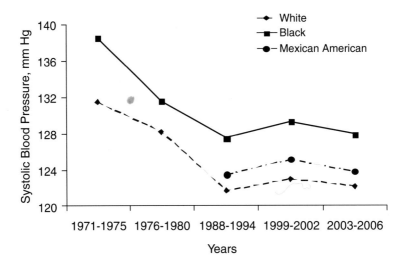

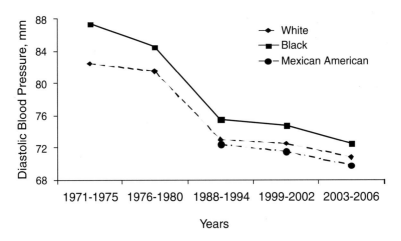

FIGURE 2-4 Age- and sex-adjusted mean systolic blood pressure (upper panel) and diastolic blood pressure (lower panel) by race or ethnicity in adults ages 20 years or older: United States, NHANES 1971-1975, 1976-1980, 1988-1994, 1999-2002, and 2003-2006.
SOURCE: CDC unpublished data.

whites and 108.9 in blacks in the NHANES 1971-1975 to 105.1 mm Hg in whites and 106.2 in blacks in the NHANES 1988-1994. Mean diastolic blood pressure decreased even more dramatically, from 68.1 mm Hg in whites and 68.1 in blacks to 57.8 mm Hg in whites and 57.3 in blacks.

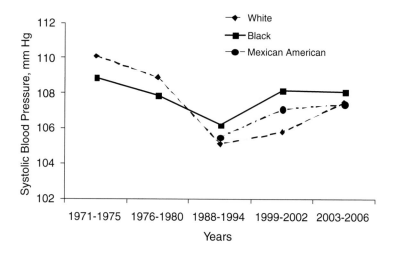

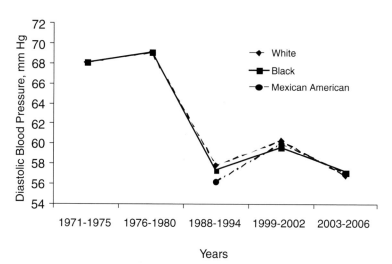

FIGURE 2-5 Age- and sex-adjusted mean systolic blood pressure and diastolic blood pressure by race or ethnicity in children ages 8-17 years: United States, NHANES 1971-1975, 1976-1980, 1988-1994, 1999-2002, and 2003-2006. SOURCE: CDC unpublished data.

During the late 1980s and the early 2000s, mean systolic blood pressure increased slightly: from 105.1, 106.2, and 105.5 mm Hg in the NHANES 1988-1994 to 107.5, 108.1, and 107.4 mm Hg in the NHANES 2003-2006 for whites, blacks, and Mexican Americans, respectively.

TRENDS IN ASSOCIATED RISK FACTORS

Overweight and obesity, high sodium intake, physical inactivity, heavy alcohol intake, low potassium intake, and a Western-style diet make up the major modifiable risk factors for hypertension (Chobanian et al., 2003; Forman et al., 2009). The literature supporting the associations between these risk factors and hypertension is well established (Chobanian et al., 2003; He et al., 2002). Thus, it is not the intent of this section to synthesize that literature but rather to comment on the direction of risk factor trends.

Risk factor data for overweight, obesity, sodium intake, and hypertension prevalence available from the National Center for Health Statistics (NCHS) *Health, United States, 2008* report show substantial increases since 1960. For example, the prevalence of obesity has increased from 13.3 to 33.4 percent between 1960-1962 and 2003-2006. Mean sodium intake increased from 2,200 to 3,500 mg per day between 1971-1974 and 1999-2000. These data are presented in Table 2-5 and Figure 2-6.

Additional data from 1998 to 2006 show that 30 to 60 percent of adults across the lifespan in the United States are physically inactive, and rates have not changed considerably over time (NCHS, 2009). Heavy drinking rates among adults ages 18 years and older have been estimated at 5 to 6 percent between 1998 and 2006 (NCHS, 2009). There has been some increase in heavy drinking among subgroups of the population ages 45-54 years and 65-74 years (NCHS, 2009).

A good source of dietary potassium can be found in fruits and vegetables. Although consumption of the recommended five servings of fruits and vegetables will not meet the recommended daily intake for potassium, it can certainly contribute (along with consumption of dairy products) to reaching that goal. Trends in fruit and vegetable consumption in the U.S. population, however, do not appear to be helping to reach that goal. In fact, trends show that the 1990 Dietary Guideline recommendations of two servings of fruit and three servings of vegetables every day are not being met. Data from the Behavioral Risk Factor Surveillance System (BRFSS) found a slight decrease in the mean frequency of fruit and vegetable consumption among men and women from 1994 to 2005 (standardized change: total, –0.22 times per day; men, –0.26 times per day; women, –0.17 times per day). From 1994 to 2005, the proportion of men and women eating fruits and vegetables or both five or more times per day remained nearly unchanged (men, 20.6 percent vs. 20.3 percent; women, 28.4 percent vs. 29.6 percent).

Kant et al. (2007) analyzed differences in diets between blacks and whites in the United States using the National Health Examination Survey data. From 1971 to 2002, black men and women reported lower intakes

TABLE 2-5 Prevalence of Hypertension (averaged measures), Overweight, Obesity, and Average Intake of Dietary Sodium per 1,000 Adults 1960-2006

	1960-1962	1971-1974	1976-1980	1988-1994	1999-2000	1999-2002	2001-2004	2003-2006
Hypertension	38.1*	39.8*	40.4*	25.5	32.8	30.0	30.9	31.3
Overweight[a]	44.8*	44.7*	47.4*	56.0	64.5	65.1	66.0	66.7
Obesity	13.3*	14.3*	15.1*	22.9	30.5	30.4	31.4	33.4
Sodium (mg/day)[b]		2,200*	2,900*	3,600*	3,500*			

[a]Includes obesity.

[b]Sodium intake estimates are based on the average of salt intake from 24-hour recalls for men and women from NHANES data. Data from NHANES 1971-1974 include naturally occurring sodium in foods and that added by processors. Data for NHANES 1999-2000 includes naturally occurring sodium in foods and that added by processors and discretionary salt usage.

*For ages 20-74, other data for ages 20 and over

SOURCES: Briefel and Johnson, 2004; NCHS, 2003, 2009, 2010.

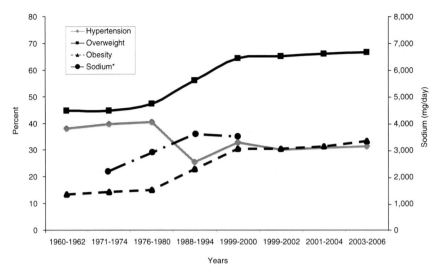

FIGURE 2-6 Secular trends in hypertension, overweight, obesity, and sodium intake in the United States.
*Sodium data from Briefel and Johnson, 2004 (note, the right y axis is in mg per day of sodium intake (e.g., 2,200 mg per day).
SOURCE: NCHS, 2003, 2009, 2010.

of vegetables, potassium, and calcium (p < 0.001) than whites (Kant et al., 2007).

In 2007, the CDC's BRFSS and the Youth Risk Behavior Surveillance System found that only 14 percent of adults and 9 percent of teens meet Healthy People 2010 goals for fruit and vegetable consumption (CDC, 2009).

RECOMMENDATIONS

Data collection is fundamental to addressing any public health problem. Data are critical for determining the burden of hypertension, characterizing the patterns among subgroups of the population, assessing changes in the problem over time, and evaluating the success of interventions. Given the challenges posed by the changing methodologies used to collect blood pressure measurements, the committee believes that efforts to strengthen hypertension surveillance and monitoring are critical.

2.1 The committee recommends that the Division for Heart Disease and Stroke Prevention (DHDSP)

- Identify methods to better use (analyze and report) existing data on the monitoring and surveillance of hypertension over time.
- Develop norms for data collection, analysis, and reporting of future surveillance of blood pressure levels and hypertension.

In developing better data collection methods and analyses, the DHDSP should increase and improve analysis and reporting of understudied populations including: children, racial and ethnic minorities, the elderly, and socioeconomic groups.

In responding to these recommendations, the DHDSP may want to consider conducting a thorough analytical assessment of available data, including data from the NHANES, to determine if these data are sufficiently comparable for evaluating secular trends of hypertension prevalence in the U.S. population. The analysis would determine at which year the data are robust enough to start analyzing secular trends, make recommendations regarding the use of less robust data, and standardize the use of appropriate age groups for reporting data so that secular trends are reported more consistently in the literature. The DHDSP may also consider conducting analysis of data on the prevalence of hypertension that account for differences in data collection methods used in NHANES (measurement on a single day, variable number of blood pressure measures taken) and the diagnosis of hypertension in clinical practice (blood pressure measurements based on at least two different days). Because of practical issues in conducting the NHANES survey, this might be done by statistical adjustment using multiple measures of blood pressure in a random sub-sample.

REFERENCES

Apostolides, A. Y., G. Cutter, S. A. Daugherty, R. Detels, J. Kraus, S. Wassertheil-Smoller, and J. Ware. 1982. Three-year incidence of hypertension in thirteen U.S. Communities. On behalf of the hypertension detection and follow-up program cooperative group. *Preventive Medicine* 11(5):487-499.

Berenson, G., S. Srinivasan, W. Chen, S. Li, D. Patel, and G. Bogalusa Heart Study. 2006. Racial (black-white) contrasts of risk for hypertensive disease in youth have implications for preventive care: The Bogalusa Heart Study. *Ethnicity & Disease* 16(3 Suppl 4):S4-2-9.

Briefel, R. R., and C. L. Johnson. 2004. Secular trends in dietary intake in the United States. *Annual Review of Nutrition* 24:401-431.

Burt, V. L., J. A. Cutler, M. Higgins, M. J. Horan, D. Labarthe, P. Whelton, C. Brown, and E. J. Roccella. 1995. Trends in the prevalence, awareness, treatment, and control of hypertension in the adult US population. Data from the health examination surveys, 1960 to 1991. *Hypertension* 26(1):60-69.

CDC (Centers for Disease Control and Prevention). 2009. *State indicator report on fruits and vegetables, 2009.* http://www.fruitsandveggiesmatter.gov/health_professionals/state report.html (accessed November 9, 2009).

Chobanian, A. V., G. L. Bakris, H. R. Black, W. C. Cushman, L. A. Green, J. L. Izzo, Jr., D. W. Jones, B. J. Materson, S. Oparil, J. T. Wright, Jr., and E. J. Roccella. 2003. The Seventh Report of the Joint National Committee on Prevention, Detection, Evaluation, and Treatment of High Blood Pressure: The JNC 7 report. *Journal of the American Medical Association* 289(19):2560-2572.

Collins, R., R. Peto, S. MacMahon, P. Hebert, N. H. Fiebach, K. A. Eberlein, J. Godwin, N. Qizilbash, J. O. Taylor, and C. H. Hennekens. 1990. Blood pressure, stroke, and coronary heart disease. Part 2, short-term reductions in blood pressure: Overview of randomised drug trials in their epidemiological context. *Lancet* 335(8693):827-838.

Cooper, R. 2009. *Hypertension and race: Origins, explanations and things we might do about it.* Washington, DC: PowerPoint presentation at Committee on Public Health Priorities to Reduce and Control Hypertension open session on June 1, 2009.

Cornoni-Huntley, J., A. Z. LaCroix, and R. J. Havlik. 1989. Race and sex differentials in the impact of hypertension in the United States. The National Health and Nutrition Examination Survey I Epidemiologic Follow-up Study. *Archives of Internal Medicine* 149(4):780-788.

Cutler, J. A., P. D. Sorlie, M. Wolz, T. Thom, L. E. Fields, and E. J. Roccella. 2008. Trends in hypertension prevalence, awareness, treatment, and control rates in United States adults between 1988-1994 and 1999-2004. *Hypertension* 52(5):818-827.

Din-Dzietham, R., Y. Liu, M.-V. Bielo, and F. Shamsa. 2007. High blood pressure trends in children and adolescents in national surveys, 1963 to 2002. [see comment]. *Circulation* 116(13):1488-1496.

Ezzati, M., A. D. Lopez, A. Rodgers, S. Vander Hoorn, and C. J. Murray. 2002. Selected major risk factors and global and regional burden of disease. *Lancet* 360(9343):1347-1360.

Falaschetti, E., M. Chaudhury, J. Mindell, and N. Poulter. 2009. Continued improvement in hypertension management in England: Results from the Health Survey for England 2006. *Hypertension* 53(3):480-486.

Fields, L. E., V. L. Burt, J. A. Cutler, J. Hughes, E. J. Roccella, and P. Sorlie. 2004. The burden of adult hypertension in the United States 1999 to 2000: A rising tide. *Hypertension* 44(4):398-404.

Forman, J. P., M. J. Stampfer, and G. C. Curhan. 2009. Diet and lifestyle risk factors associated with incident hypertension in women. *Journal of the American Medical Association* 302(4):401-411.

Fuchs, F. D., L. E. Chambless, P. K. Whelton, F. J. Nieto, and G. Heiss. 2001. Alcohol consumption and the incidence of hypertension: The Atherosclerosis Risk in Communities Study. *Hypertension* 37(5):1242-1250.

Gaziano, T. A., A. Bitton, S. Anand, and M. C. Weinstein. 2009. The global cost of nonoptimal blood pressure. *Journal of Hypertension* 27(7):1472-1477.

Gregg, E. W., Y. J. Cheng, B. L. Cadwell, G. Imperatore, D. E. Williams, K. M. Flegal, K. M. Narayan, and D. F. Williamson. 2005. Secular trends in cardiovascular disease risk factors according to body mass index in US adults. *Journal of the American Medical Association* 293(15):1868-1874.

Gu, D., K. Reynolds, X. Wu, J. Chen, X. Duan, P. Muntner, G. Huang, R. F. Reynolds, S. Su, P. K. Whelton, and J. He. 2002. Prevalence, awareness, treatment, and control of hypertension in China. *Hypertension* 40(6):920-927.

Gu, D., T. N. Kelly, X. Wu, J. Chen, X. Duan, J. F. Huang, J. C. Chen, P. K. Whelton, and J. He. 2008. Blood pressure and risk of cardiovascular disease in Chinese men and women. *American Journal of Hypertension* 21(3):265-272.

Hajjar, I., and T. A. Kotchen. 2003. Trends in prevalence, awareness, treatment, and control of hypertension in the United States, 1988-2000. [see comment]. *Journal of the American Medical Association* 290(2):199-206.

He, J., P. Muntner, J. Chen, E. J. Roccella, R. H. Streiffer, and P. K. Whelton. 2002. Factors associated with hypertension control in the general population of the United States. *Archives of Internal Medicine* 162(9):1051-1058.

He, J., P. M. Kearney, and P. Muntner. 2003. Blood pressure and risk of vascular disease. In *Lifestyle Modification for the Prevention and Treatment of Hypertension,* edited by P. K. Whelton, J. He, and G. T. Louis. New York: Marcel Dekker, Inc. Pp. 23-52.

Hebert, P. R., M. Moser, J. Mayer, R. J. Glynn, and C. H. Hennekens. 1993. Recent evidence on drug therapy of mild to moderate hypertension and decreased risk of coronary heart disease. *Archives of Internal Medicine* 153(5):578-581.

Hyman, D. J., and V. N. Pavlik. 2001. Characteristics of patients with uncontrolled hypertension in the United States. [see comment] [erratum appears in 2002 *New England Journal of Medicine* 346(7):544]. *New England Journal of Medicine* 345(7):479-486.

Joffres, M. R., P. Ghadirian, J. G. Fodor, A. Petrasovits, A. Chockalingam, and P. Hamet. 1997. Awareness, treatment, and control of hypertension in Canada. *American Journal of Hypertension* 10(10 Pt 1):1097-1102.

Kannel, W. B. 1996. Blood pressure as a cardiovascular risk factor: Prevention and treatment. *Journal of the American Medical Association* 275(20):1571-1576.

Kant, A. K., B. I. Graubard, and S. K. Kumanyika. 2007. Trends in black-white differentials in dietary intakes of U.S. adults, 1971-2002. *American Journal of Preventive Medicine* 32(4):264-272.

Kearney, P. M., M. Whelton, K. Reynolds, P. Muntner, P. K. Whelton, and J. He. 2005. Global burden of hypertension: Analysis of worldwide data. *Lancet* 365(9455):217-223.

Klag, M. J., P. K. Whelton, B. L. Randall, J. D. Neaton, F. L. Brancati, C. E. Ford, N. B. Shulman, and J. Stamler. 1996. Blood pressure and end-stage renal disease in men. *New England Journal of Medicine* 334(1):13-18.

Lawes, C. M., S. Vander Hoorn, and A. Rodgers. 2008. Global burden of blood-pressure-related disease, 2001. *Lancet* 371(9623):1513-1518.

Lewington, S., R. Clarke, N. Qizilbash, R. Peto, and R. Collins. 2002. Age-specific relevance of usual blood pressure to vascular mortality: A meta-analysis of individual data for one million adults in 61 prospective studies. *Lancet* 360(9349):1903-1913.

Lloyd-Jones, D., R. Adams, M. Carnethon, G. De Simone, T. B. Ferguson, K. Flegal, E. Ford, K. Furie, A. Go, K. Greenlund, N. Haase, S. Hailpern, M. Ho, V. Howard, B. Kissela, S. Kittner, D. Lackland, L. Lisabeth, A. Marelli, M. McDermott, J. Meigs, D. Mozaffarian, G. Nichol, C. O'Donnell, V. Roger, W. Rosamond, R. Sacco, P. Sorlie, R. Stafford, J. Steinberger, T. Thom, S. Wasserthiel-Smoller, N. Wong, J. Wylie-Rosett, and Y. Hong. 2009. Heart disease and stroke statistics—2009 update: A report from the American Heart Association Statistics Committee and Stroke Statistics subcommittee. *Circulation* 119(3):480-486.

MacMahon, S., R. Peto, J. Cutler, R. Collins, P. Sorlie, J. Neaton, R. Abbott, J. Godwin, A. Dyer, and J. Stamler. 1990. Blood pressure, stroke, and coronary heart disease. Part 1, prolonged differences in blood pressure: Prospective observational studies corrected for the regression dilution bias. *Lancet* 335(8692):765-774.

Manolio, T. A., G. L. Burke, P. J. Savage, S. Sidney, J. M. Gardin, and A. Oberman. 1994. Exercise blood pressure response and 5-year risk of elevated blood pressure in a cohort of young adults: The CARDIA study. *American Journal of Hypertension* 7(3):234-241.

Muntner, P., J. He, J. A. Cutler, R. P. Wildman, and P. K. Whelton. 2004. Trends in blood pressure among children and adolescents. *Journal of the American Medical Association* 291(17):2107-2113.

National High Blood Pressure Education Program Working Group on High Blood Pressure in Children and Adolescents. 2004. The fourth report on the diagnosis, evaluation, and treatment of high blood pressure in children and adolescents. [see comment]. *Pediatrics* 114(2 Suppl 4):555-576.

NCHS (National Center for Health Statistics). 2003. *Health, United States, 2003 with chartbook on trends in the health of Americans.* Hyattsville, MD: National Center for Health Statistics.

———. 2009. *Health, United States, 2008* with special feature on the health of young adults. Hyattsville, MD: National Center for Health Statistics.

———. 2010. *Health, United States, 2009 with special feature on medical technology.* Hyattsville, MD: National Center for Health Statistics.

Ostchega, Y., C. F. Dillon, J. P. Hughes, M. Carroll, and S. Yoon. 2007. Trends in hypertension prevalence, awareness, treatment, and control in older U.S. adults: Data from the National Health and Nutrition Examination Survey 1988 to 2004. *Journal of the American Geriatrics Society* 55(7):1056-1065.

Ostchega, Y., M. Carroll, R. J. Prineas, M. A. McDowell, T. Louis, and T. Tilert. 2009. Trends of elevated blood pressure among children and adolescents: Data from the National Health and Nutrition Examination Survey 1988-2006. *American Journal of Hypertension* 22(1):59-67.

Pickering, T. G., J. E. Hall, L. J. Appel, B. E. Falkner, J. Graves, M. N. Hill, D. W. Jones, T. Kurtz, S. G. Sheps, and E. J. Roccella. 2005. Recommendations for blood pressure measurement in humans and experimental animals: Part 1: Blood pressure measurement in humans: A statement for professionals from the Subcommittee of Professional and Public Education of the American Heart Association Council on High Blood Pressure Research. *Circulation* 111(5):697-716.

Staessen, J. A., J. G. Wang, and L. Thijs. 2001. Cardiovascular protection and blood pressure reduction: A meta-analysis. *Lancet* 358(9290):1305-1315.

Stamler, J., R. Stamler, and J. D. Neaton. 1993. Blood pressure, systolic and diastolic, and cardiovascular risks. US population data. *Archives of Internal Medicine* 153(5):598-615.

Vasan, R. S., A. Beiser, S. Seshadri, M. G. Larson, W. B. Kannel, R. B. D'Agostino, and D. Levy. 2002. Residual lifetime risk for developing hypertension in middle-aged women and men: The Framingham Heart Study. *Journal of the American Medical Association* 287(8):1003-1010.

Wang, T. J., and R. S. Vasan. 2005. Epidemiology of uncontrolled hypertension in the United States. *Circulation* 112(11):1651-1662.

Whelton, P. K. 1994. Epidemiology of hypertension. *Lancet* 344(8915):101-106.

Wu, Y., R. Huxley, L. Li, V. Anna, G. Xie, C. Yao, M. Woodward, X. Li, J. Chalmers, R. Gao, L. Kong, X. Yang, N. S. C. China, and N. W. G. China. 2008. Prevalence, awareness, treatment, and control of hypertension in China: Data from the China National Nutrition and Health Survey 2002. *Circulation* 118(25):2679-2686.

3

The Role of the Division for Heart Disease and Stroke Prevention in the Prevention and Control of Hypertension

Critical to any organization is its capacity to achieve its mission and goals; thus, the resources available and the authority it has to address its charge are fundamental to its ability to act. This chapter provides a brief overview of the Centers for Disease Control and Prevention's (CDC's) Division for Heart Disease and Stroke Prevention, its resources, the legislative history of relevant programs, and an overview of activities directed at preventing and reducing hypertension in the United States.

The Cardiovascular Health Studies Branch, established in 1989 within the Division of Adult and Community Health in the National Center for Chronic Disease Prevention and Health Promotion (NCCDPHP), was the focal point for limited cardiovascular prevention and control activities at the CDC. Over the ensuing 17 years, the CDC's activities in this area grew in part as a result of the increasing concern about the growing burden of cardiovascular disease and congressional action that provided the CDC with funds to improve the cardiovascular health of Americans. Today, cardiovascular disease prevention and control activities are under the purview of the Division for Heart Disease and Stroke Prevention (DHDSP). The charge of the division is to lead the nation's cardiovascular health initiatives and to reduce the burden of disparities associated with heart disease and stroke. The DHDSP's core functions include programs, surveillance, research, evaluation, and partnerships. Its activities are distributed among four primary programs: (1) the National Heart Disease and Stroke Prevention Program, (2) WISEWOMAN, (3) the Paul Coverdell National Acute Stroke Registry, and (4) the State Cardiovascular Health Examination Survey. Although not listed as a specific program, Congress directed the

TABLE 3-1 DHDSP Administrative and Program Budgets (FY 2008)

Core Function	Administrative Budget	Percentage of Total Administrative Budget
Programs	$49,259,915	74%
Surveillance	$5,672,580	8%
Research	$3,915,689	6%
Evaluation	$4,155,207	6%
Partnerships	$3,862,683	6%

Programs	Program Budget	Percentage of Total Program Budget
State Heart Disease and Stroke Prevention Program	$27,770,783	56%
WISEWOMAN	$15,499,336	32%
Paul Coverdell National Acute Stroke Registry	$4,400,000	9%
State Cardiovascular Health Examination Survey	$399,751	1%
Other	$1,190,045	2%

DHDSP to address sodium reduction in the American diet, but it did not appropriate funding for this activity.

PROGRAMMATIC FUNDING

In 1998, the DHDSP budget was $10.7 million. Its budget increased gradually to about $44 million in 2005 and remained relatively constant until 2008 when the budget increased to about $50 million. The DHDSP budget appropriated for fiscal year (FY) 2009 was approximately $54 million. The division's administrative budget is divided among five core functions, which are listed in Table 3-1 with their respective budgets; program expenditures, which represent almost 75 percent of the DHDSP budget, are also itemized. The budget distribution shown is for FY 2008 because the final resource allocation for 2009 had not been determined at the time of this writing.

NATIONAL HEART DISEASE AND STROKE PREVENTION PROGRAM

Established in 1998, the State Heart Disease and Stroke Prevention Program is the division's largest program. The program funds or provides tools, guidance, and other assistance to all 50 states; thus, it is now referred to as a national program. While there is no specific language authorizing the program, funds are appropriated each year in the Labor, Health and Human Service appropriations bill (or in continuing appropriations resolutions). The program was initially established in response to congressional concern that nearly 1 million Americans were dying each year from cardiovascular disease and the knowledge that the major risk factors for cardiovascular disease were modifiable and often preventable. Of further concern was that states did not receive specific federal funds, and many states had limited resources to dedicate to the prevention of cardiovascular disease. The congressional vision was that of an integrated, comprehensive, and nationwide program to provide assistance to states; support research, surveillance, and laboratory capacity; and reduce risk factors for cardiovascular disease by promoting healthy behaviors. The program was to give priority to those states with the highest age-adjusted death rates due to cardiovascular disease. To carry out this responsibility, Congress appropriated $8.1 million to the CDC for the program.

Currently the program provides funds to state health departments in 41 states and the District of Columbia. The six primary program priorities are to (1) control high blood pressure, (2) control high cholesterol, (3) improve emergency response, (4) improve the quality of care, (5) increase awareness of the signs and symptoms of heart attack and stroke and of the need to call 9-1-1, and (6) eliminate health disparities related to heart disease and stroke. Within these broad priorities, states are encouraged to focus on policy and system change, effect population-based change, ensure cultural competency, engage partners, and work within the health care, worksite, and community settings.

Under the program, states can be funded at the level of Capacity Building or Basic Implementation. Twenty-eight states receive $300,000 annually at the Capacity Building level. Their priorities include increasing collaboration between public and private partners, defining the existing burden of heart disease and stroke in the state, assessing ongoing population-based interventions, and developing a comprehensive state plan. There is also an emphasis on identifying culturally appropriate approaches to raise awareness and promote healthy behaviors. Fourteen states receive Basic Implementation funding in the amount of $1 million dollars annually. These states implement and evaluate policies, offer environmental and educational interventions in various settings, and facilitate provider education and training.

In an effort to assist in the outcome evaluation of heart disease and stroke prevention activities within states, the DHDSP developed policy and systems outcome indicators for controlling high blood pressure. State HDSP programs may use these indicators to support the development of an evaluation plan. The Logic Model for Strategies and Interventions to Reduce High Blood Pressure (Figure 3-1) provides parameters for effec-

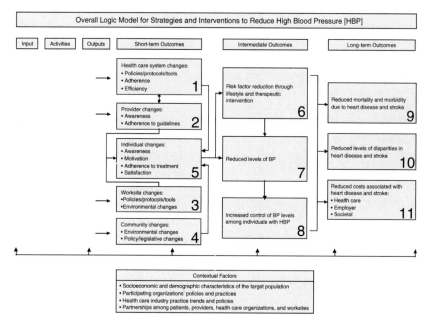

FIGURE 3-1 Overall logic model for strategies and interventions to reduce high blood pressure (HBP).
SOURCE: Ladd et al., 2010.

tive intervention strategies. Each high blood pressure control outcome indicator identified in the DHDSP's draft document can be nested within a component outlined in the logic model. The model includes a spectrum of intervention approaches, including health care system changes, provider changes, individual changes, worksite changes, and community changes, that can effectively reduce the burden of risk factors and disease.

State programs decide where along the logic model they will focus their program efforts and resources. The committee did not attempt to conduct a systematic review of state programs; however, based on a highlight of state activities provided by the DHDSP, many states tend to focus on secondary prevention activities. Such activities include improving the quality of care for individuals through clinical performance measurement (North Carolina, Utah), education and training of health care providers (Georgia, South Carolina, Virginia), and worksite wellness programs (Kansas, Maine, Missouri). Some primary and secondary prevention activities are addressed through programs that increase awareness and educate about risk factors and lifestyle changes (Oregon).

WISEWOMAN (WELL-INTEGRATED SCREENING AND EVALUATION FOR WOMEN ACROSS THE NATION)

Congress, through the Breast and Cervical Cancer Mortality Prevention Act of 1990 (Public Law 101-354) provided the authority and funding for the CDC's National Breast and Cervical Cancer Early Detection Program and the WISEWOMAN program. The WISEWOMAN provision allowed for:

> (a) Demonstration projects. In the case of States receiving grants under section 1501 [42 U.S.C. § 300k], the Secretary, acting through the Director of the Centers for Disease Control and Prevention, may make grants to not more than 3 such States to carry out demonstration projects for the purpose of– (1) providing preventive health services in addition to the services authorized in such section, including screenings regarding blood pressure and cholesterol, and including health education; (2) providing appropriate referrals for medical treatment of women receiving services pursuant to paragraph (1) and ensuring, to the extent practicable, the provision of appropriate follow-up services; and (3) evaluating activities conducted under paragraphs (1) and (2) through appropriate surveillance or program-monitoring activities.

The legislation specifically required that grants for the program be provided only through entities that screen women for breast or cervical cancer through the National Breast and Cervical Cancer Early Detection Program. As the name of the program suggests, the legislation integrates and leverages the services and efforts of a cancer screening and evaluation program with a primary prevention program to reduce cardiovascular risk in women.

The program was initially funded in 1996 at the amount of $3 million and was situated in the Division of Nutrition, Physical Activity and Obesity; in 1998, the program was transferred to DHDSP. By FY 2009, the budget had increased to $19.5 million, with an average of $600,000 dedicated to each of the 21 programs operating throughout the United States. Of WISEWOMAN funding, 80 percent is directed to programs, and within that amount, 60 percent is allocated to primary prevention through screening for hypertension, cholesterol, and (more recently) diabetes. The remaining 40 percent of funding is directed to administration, data collection, and evaluation.

The WISEWOMAN program provides screening and lifestyle interventions to low-income, uninsured, or underinsured woman between the ages of 40 and 64. WISEWOMAN has reached more than 84,000 women in need since the year 2000, providing approximately 149,000 health screenings and 210,500 lifestyle interventions through its 21 state and tribal programs. More than 7,674 new cases of hypertension have been identi-fied through WISEWOMAN screenings, as well as 7,928 cases of high cholesterol and 1,140 cases of diabetes. Women who participated in WISE-WOMAN are reportedly more likely to return for regular health screenings. A recent review of 14 WISEWOMAN programs found that the average reduction in systolic blood pressure after 1 year was 2.7 mm Hg, although it ranged from an increase of 5.0 mm Hg to a decrease of 8.0 mm Hg in the programs studied (Farris et al., 2007).

The Nebraska WISEWOMAN program was highlighted by Secretary of Health and Human Services Dr. Kathleen Sebelius in a recent report describing health care success stories. She observed that 19,000 women have been reached in Nebraska alone, helping to reduce their risk of heart attack and stroke. Dr. Sebelius encouraged building on the success of the WISEWOMAN program, which she said has provided evidence of the importance and success of prevention programs (Montz and Seshamani, 2009).

THE PAUL COVERDELL NATIONAL ACUTE STROKE REGISTRY

The CDC's effort to create state-based stroke registries was initiated in 2001 as a result of congressional language in the CDC Heart Disease and Stroke appropriations budget line. The program is also included in FY 2002-2005 appropriations; since then, no specific congressional language regarding the program has been included in appropriations, but the CDC has maintained funding for the program through the appropriations for Heart Disease and Stroke. Through the initial legislative language, Con-gress awarded the CDC $4.5 million to track and improve the delivery of care to patients with acute stroke. As a first step, the CDC was to consult with stroke organizations and others to develop specific data elements for a stroke registry and to design and pilot registry prototypes. The focus of the registry data collection effort was to measure the quality of care deliv-ered to stroke patients from emergency response to hospital care. Between 2001 and 2002, eight states participated in piloting prototype projects (California, Georgia, Illinois, Massachusetts, Michigan, North Carolina, Ohio, and Oregon). Results from these pilot projects revealed disparities between generally recommended standards for treating stroke patients and actual hospital practices. In 2004, four of the pilot states were funded to establish statewide registries (Georgia, Illinois, Massachusetts, and North Carolina) to collect and analyze data and implement quality improvement interventions at the hospital level. In 2007, funding was extended to six state health departments (Georgia, Massachusetts, Michigan, Minnesota, North Carolina, and Ohio) for a new 5-year period. In that same year, the CDC, along with The Joint Commission's Primary Stroke Center Certification Program and the American Stroke Association's (a division of the American Heart Association) Get with the Guidelines Stroke Program, formed an agreement to jointly release a set of standardized stroke performance measures. These guidelines are intended to foster collaboration and encourage hospital participation.

STATE CARDIOVASCULAR HEALTH EXAMINATION SURVEY

The State Cardiovascular Health Examination Survey was initiated in 2005 in an attempt to advance state capacity in the development of hypertension and cholesterol control strategies. A Heart Disease and Stroke Prevention Program funding opportunity announcement provided the initial funding, but the program now has its own funding opportunity announcement. States must receive funding from the DHDSP as a prerequisite to receiving state cardiovascular health examination funds. Three state health departments (Arkansas, Kansas, and Washington) were the initial awardees; Oklahoma was added in 2007. State awardees design a survey to collect data on blood pressure, cholesterol, and other relevant cardiovascular health information, including risk factors and health behaviors. The goal of the program is to provide data with which to monitor progress toward the Healthy People 2010 objectives related to control of high blood pressure and high cholesterol.

ACTIVITIES TO REDUCE SODIUM INTAKE

Congress, through the Omnibus Appropriations Act (Public Law 111-8) in the Joint Explanatory Statement: Division F—Labor, Health and Human Services, and Education, and Related Agencies Appropriations, 2009, included an unfunded mandate for the CDC to engage in activities to reduce sodium. The statement specifically states:

> A diet high in sodium is a major cause of heart disease and stroke. CDC is encouraged to work with major food manufacturers and chain restaurants to reduce sodium levels in their products. The agency is directed to submit to the Committees on Appropriations and the House of Representatives and the Senate an evaluation of its sodium-reduction activities by no later than 15 months after the enactment of this Act, and annually thereafter.

In January 2009, the DHDSP and the National Heart, Lung, and Blood Institute (NHLBI) commissioned the Food and Nutrition Board of the Institute of Medicine (IOM) to form an ad hoc Committee on Strategies to Reduce Sodium Intake. The committee is cosponsored by the Health and Human Services' Food and Drug Administration and the Office of Disease Prevention and Health Promotion (Office of Public Health and Science,

Office of the Secretary). The committee is tasked with identifying means to reduce dietary sodium intake to levels recommended by the Dietary Guidelines for Americans (HHS and USDA, 2005). A range of approaches will be reviewed, including regulatory and legislative actions, new product development, and food reformulation, as well as public health and educational interventions. Opportunities to foster collaborations among industry, government, and the health care enterprise will be considered. The anticipated publication date of the consensus report is early 2010.

OTHER PROGRAMMATIC ACTIVITIES

Healthy People

The DHDSP, along with the National Institutes of Health (NIH), is responsible for monitoring progress toward reaching Healthy People goals related to cardiovascular health. Healthy People is a national prevention agenda that was first articulated in 1979 by the Department of Health, Education, and Welfare through *Healthy People: The Surgeon General's Report on Health Promotion and Disease Prevention* (DHEW, 1979). The IOM and the 1978 Departmental Task Force on Disease Prevention and Health Promotion contributed to its preparation. The report's central theme emphasized the role of individuals, as well as public and private sector decision makers, in promoting healthier lifestyles. Blood pressure screening, along with the elimination of cigarette smoking and dietary changes to reduce intake of excess calories, fat, salt, and sugar, were identified as health-enhancing measures "within the practical grasp of most Americans." The reduction of heart attacks and strokes was a subgoal identified in the report's section dedicated to healthy adults. Increased efforts in "preventive measures such as high blood pressure detection and control, reduction of smoking, prudent diet, increased exercise and fitness, and better stress management" were suggested strategies in working toward this subgoal. *Promoting Health/Preventing Disease: Objectives for the Nation* (HHS, 1980) was released as a companion to this report in 1980; it identified 226 specific, measurable, health objectives and strategies for achieving them.

Healthy People 2000 (HHS, 1991), released in 1990, set forth 22 priority areas, including one on heart disease and stroke (Priority Area 15). At that time, the NHLBI was designated as the lead agency assigned to this area. The objectives identified in this area included the reduction of coronary heart disease and stroke deaths and also addressed cholesterol, smoking, dietary fat, physical activity, and overweight. The objectives relating to hypertension included efforts to increase control of high blood pressure, increase therapeutic actions by those with high blood pressure, and increase blood pressure screening.

Released in 2000, the *Healthy People 2010* (HHS, 2000a,b) report builds on *Healthy People 2000*. It consolidated 16 objectives for heart disease and stroke prevention into one section (Focus Area 12). The CDC joined with the NHLBI to co-lead and share accountability for progress toward achieving these objectives. The following objectives relate specifically to hypertension:

- Reduce the proportion of adults with high blood pressure.
- Increase the proportion of adults with high blood pressure whose blood pressure is under control.
- Increase the proportion of adults with high blood pressure who are taking action (for example, losing weight, increasing physical activity, and reducing sodium intake) to help control their blood pressure.
- Increase the proportion of adults who have had their blood pressure measured within the preceding two years and can state whether their blood pressure was normal or high.
- Increase the proportion of persons aged 2 years and older who consume 2,400 mg or less of sodium daily.

Other partners engaged in working with the DHDSP and NHLBI to achieve these goals included other CDC units, other federal agencies, and the American Heart Association. The Memorandum of Understanding signed by these partners in 2001 created the Healthy People 2010 Partnership for Heart Disease and Stroke Prevention, which in 2003 became the National Forum for Heart Disease and Stroke Prevention and includes a much broader array of participants. The Partnership/Forum began charting a public health action plan to work toward achieving the Healthy People goals. The action plan follows later in this section.

The *Healthy People 2010 Midcourse Review* (HHS, 2006) assessed progress toward the 10 (out of 16) objectives related to heart disease and stroke for which data were available. The results are summarized in Figure 3-2.

The problem of hypertension is addressed in the following paragraphs:

... prevalence of high blood pressure is cause for serious concern. The baseline level was 26% and the target is 14%. On the basis of the same NHANES [National Health and Nutrition Examination Survey] sources as cholesterol levels, prevalence of high blood pressure increased by 33% of the target change as of 1999-2002, a change in prevalence from 26% to approximately 30% among adults aged 20 years or older. This change, coupled with the striking increase in prevalence of diabetes and obesity, adds to the total cardiovascular disease burden and threatens to slow progress toward the goals for heart disease and stroke mortality through the remainder of the decade.

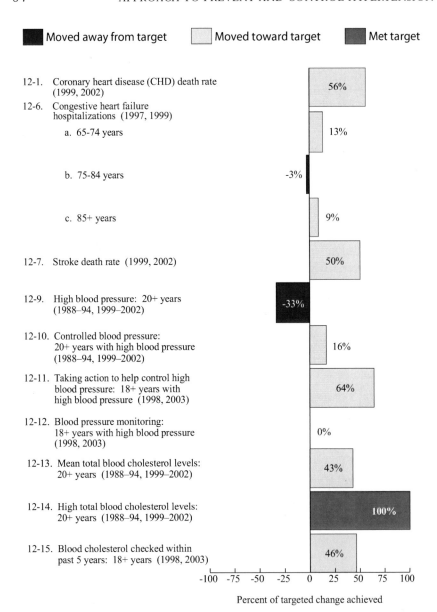

FIGURE 3-2 Progress quotient chart for Healthy People 2010 Focus Area 12: Heart Disease and Stroke.
SOURCE: HHS, 2006.

> Adding to concern about the nation's course with respect to high blood pressure is the report of increasing blood pressure among children and adolescents from 1988-1994 to 1999-2000. . . . During this period, the national population mean levels of systolic and diastolic blood pressure increased for each of two age groups, 8-12 and 13-17 years. Increases were greatest for non-Hispanic blacks and Mexican Americans and reached +4.8 mm/Hg overall for those aged 8-12 years. These increases were only partially accounted for by the concurrent increase in body mass index. (HHS, 2008, p. 34)

Clearly, there is concern that the increasing prevalence of high blood pressure in adults and increasing blood pressure levels in children is moving in the wrong direction from the specified goals.

A Public Health Action Plan to Prevent Heart Disease and Stroke

The DHDSP, as a co-lead partner in the National Forum for Heart Disease and Stroke Prevention, initiated the development of the *Public Health Action Plan to Prevent Heart Disease and Stroke* (HHS, 2003). It was responsible for overall planning and execution and for coordinating input from partners, working groups, and expert panels. The resulting Action Plan, issued in 2003 and updated in 2008, was viewed as a "call to action for tackling one our nation's foremost challenges, to prevent and control chronic diseases" (HHS, 2003, p. v). The plan provides a vision for the future and a framework of action for public health practitioners and policy makers in the areas of preventing the development of risk factors for heart disease and stroke; detecting and treating risk factors; achieving early identification and treatment of cardiovascular disease and stroke, especially in the acute phases; and preventing the recurrence and complications of heart disease and stroke.

The Action Plan is not specific to the prevention and control of hypertension; rather, it is written for the most part in the general terms of preventing heart disease and stroke. Two recommendations were considered fundamental to the plan:

Effective Communication:
- The urgency and promise of preventing heart disease and stroke and their precursors (i.e., atherosclerosis, high blood pressure, and their risk factors and determinants) must be communicated effectively by the public health community through a new long-term strategy of public information and education. This new strategy must engage national, state, and local policy makers and other stakeholders. (Revised in 2008 to include: As a matter of emphasis,

special consideration must be paid to those most at risk. Communication strategies should utilize the most current forms of available technology as well at those communication devices that are accessible in various communities in the United States and globally.)

Strategic Leadership, Partnership, and Organization:
- The nations' public health agencies and their partners (revised in 2008 to include: and the public) must provide the necessary leadership for a comprehensive public health strategy to prevent heart disease and stroke. (HHS, 2008)

Among the remaining 22 recommendations, two included direct reference to blood pressure.

Advancing Policy: Defining the Issues and Finding the Needed Solutions:
- Conduct and facilitate research by means of collaboration among interested parties to identify new policy, environmental, and sociocultural priorities for CVH [cardiovascular health] promotion. Once the priorities are identified, determine the best methods for translating, disseminating, and sustaining them. Fund research to identify barriers and effective interventions in order to translate science into practice and thereby improve access to and use of quality health care and improve outcomes for patients with or at risk for CVD [cardiovascular disease]. Conduct economics research, including cost-effectiveness studies and comprehensive economic models that assess the return on investment for CVH promotion as well as primary and secondary CVD prevention.

As an example, research to assess community-wide interventions aimed at maintaining and restoring low blood cholesterol levels and low blood pressure, which help prevent atherosclerosis and high blood pressure, are suggested. This recommendation was designated a 2008-2009 priority.

- Design, plan, implement, and evaluate a comprehensive intervention for children and youth in school, family, and community settings. This intervention must address dietary imbalances, physical inactivity, tobacco use, and other determinants in order to prevent development of risk factors and progression of atherosclerosis and high blood pressure.

A full list of the updated 22 recommendations is included in Appendix C.

DIVISION FOR HEART DISEASE AND STROKE PREVENTION STRATEGIC PLAN

The DHDSP's Strategic Plan is modeled on the Healthy People 2010 goals related to heart disease and stroke and the recommendations set forth in *A Public Health Action Plan to Prevent Heart Disease and Stroke* (HHS, 2003). The division is focused on efforts to (1) prevent risk factors for heart disease and stroke; (2) increase detection and treatment of risk factors; (3) increase detection and treatment of heart disease and stroke; (4) decrease recurrences of heart disease and stroke; and (5) foster a skilled and engaged public health workforce (Appendix D). Several priority areas were identified as areas of emphasis over the course of the next several years. The first priority is the enhancement of collaboration by the CDC with federal, state, and local agencies and with nongovernmental organizations to mobilize prevention efforts. The division will also prioritize efforts to identify and address at-risk populations to prevent disparities associated with heart disease and stroke. An internal Disparities Workgroup was formed in 2007 in support of this effort.

DHDSP COLLABORATION WITH OTHER CDC UNITS

Many of the DHDSP's programmatic efforts focus on secondary prevention of heart disease and stroke with limited primary prevention activities. Some of the relevant primary prevention activities are the domain of other divisions of the National Coordinating Center for Chronic Disease Prevention and Health Promotion that focus broadly on preventing chronic diseases and their risk factors. These divisions work as separate organizational units, each with its own budget and mission related to a specific disease, risk factor(s), or vulnerable population. Some of these units also address adolescents and young adults.

According to division staff, the DHDSP maintains an ongoing working relationship with its sister divisions and will collaborate on relevant efforts. Table 3-2 lists FY 2009 funding and program descriptions for CDC units with which the DHDSP collaborates.

For example, the DHDSP leads the Cardiovascular Health Collaboration, a monthly meeting of NCCDPHP division leadership and representatives from other CDC centers to discuss important and timely cardiovascular health-related issues. The DHDSP collaborated with the Office on Smoking and Health (OSH) on an IOM report about the effects of secondhand smoke and acute cardiac events and connected the WISEWOMAN programs with tobacco quit lines. As noted earlier, the DHDSP is also working with the Division of Nutrition, Physical Activity, and Obesity on an IOM consensus study to identify strategies for reducing sodium in the food supply as well as a broader salt initiative and related issues such as menu labeling.

TABLE 3-2 CDC Units or Programs, Funding and Program Description

CDC Unit or Program	FY 2009 Funding (millions)	Program Description
Division for Heart Disease and Stroke Prevention (DHDSP)	$54.1	
Division of Adolescent and School Health (DASH)	$57.6	DASH funds education and health agencies in 22 states and 1 tribal government to help schools implement a coordinated school health approach, with an emphasis on promoting physical activity, healthy eating, and a tobacco-free lifestyle. The CDC also funds 50 state education agencies (including the District of Columbia), 1 tribal government, 6 territorial education agencies, and 16 large urban school districts for school-based HIV prevention. Ten large urban school districts receive CDC support for school-based asthma management programs.
Division of Nutrition, Physical Activity, and Obesity (DNPAO)	$44.3	DNPAO funds health departments in 23 states to coordinate statewide efforts with multiple partners to address obesity. The program's focus is on policy and environmental change initiatives directed toward increasing physical activity; consumption of fruits and vegetables; breastfeeding initiation, duration, and exclusivity; and decreasing television viewing and consumption of sugar-sweetened beverages and high-energy-dense foods (foods high in calories).
Division of Adult and Community Health (DACH)		
Racial and Ethnic Approaches to Community Health (REACH)	$35.6	REACH supports community coalitions that design, implement, evaluate, and disseminate community-driven strategies to eliminate health disparities in key areas. REACH supports the CDC's strategic goals by addressing health disparities throughout infancy, childhood, adolescence, adulthood, and older adulthood. This program has developed innovative approaches that focus on racial and ethnic groups and is improving people's health in communities, health care settings, schools, and work sites.

TABLE 3-2 Continued

CDC Unit or Program	FY 2009 Funding (millions)	Program Description
Healthy Communities	$22.8	DACH currently provides guidance, technical assistance, and training to 12 Strategic Alliance for Health communities selected to represent a mix of urban, rural, and tribal communities. DACH will also train and support more than 200 ACHIEVE (Action Communities for Health, Innovation, and Environmental Change) communities over the next several years. ACHIEVE selects communities to participate in an Action Institute, which convenes community action teams and trains community leaders making policy, systems, and environmental changes to prevent and control chronic diseases and their risk factors. DACH also supports the YMCA of the Pioneering Healthier Communities initiative.
Preventive Health and Health Services (PHHS) Block Grant	$102.0	The PHHS block grant provides funding for all 50 states, the District of Columbia, 2 tribes, and 8 territories to tailor prevention and health promotion programs to their particular public health needs. The block grant gives its grantees the flexibility to target funds to prevent and control chronic diseases such as heart disease, diabetes, and arthritis and helps them to respond quickly to outbreaks of food-borne infections and waterborne diseases.
Prevention Research Centers (PRCs)	$31.1	The CDC supports 33 centers associated with schools of public health or medicine throughout the country. Each center conducts at least one core research project with an underserved population that has a disproportionately large burden of disease and disability. All centers share a common goal of addressing behaviors and environmental factors that contribute to chronic diseases such as cancer, heart disease, and diabetes. Several PRCs also address injury, infectious disease, mental health, oral health, and global health.
Office on Smoking and Health (OSH)	$106.2	OSH funds programs in all 50 states, the District of Columbia, 8 territories or jurisdictions, and 7 tribal-serving organizations. In addition, the CDC funds national networks to reduce tobacco use among specific populations. The CDC also provides funding to 22 state education agencies and 1 tribal government for coordinated school health programs to help prevent tobacco use.

SOURCE: Personal communication, D. Labarthe, Centers for Disease Control and Prevention, May 15, 2009.

REFERENCES

DHEW (Department of Health, Education, and Welfare). 1979. *Healthy people: The Surgeon General's report on health promotion and disease prevention.* Washington, DC: U.S. Government Printing Office.

Farris, R. P., J. C. Will, O. Khavjou, and E. A. Finkelstein. 2007. Beyond effectiveness: Evaluating the public health impact of the WISEWOMAN program. *American Journal of Public Health* 97(4):641-647.

HHS (U.S. Department of Health and Human Services). 1980. *Promoting health/preventing disease: Objectives for the nation.* Washington, DC: Public Health Service.

———. 1991. *Healthy people 2000: National health promotion and disease prevention objectives.* Rockville, MD: Public Health Service.

———. 2000a. *Healthy People 2010,* 2nd ed. Vol. 1. Washington, DC: U.S. Government Printing Office.

———. 2000b. *Healthy People 2010,* 2nd ed. Vol. 2. Washington, DC: U.S. Government Printing Office.

———. 2003. *A Public Health Action Plan to prevent heart disease and stroke.* Atlanta, GA: U.S. Department of Health and Human Services, Centers for Disease Control and Prevention.

———. 2006. *Healthy People 2010 midcourse review.* Washington, DC: U.S. Government Printing Office.

———. 2008. *2008 Public Health Action Plan update: Celebrating our first five years.* Atlanta, GA: U.S. Department of Health and Human Services, Centers for Disease Control and Prevention.

HHS and USDA (U.S. Department of Agriculture). 2005. *Dietary guidelines for Americans.* 6th ed. Washington, DC: U.S. Government Printing Office.

Ladd, S., H. Wall, T. Rogers, E. Fulmer, K. Leeks, S. Lim, and J. Jernigan. 2010. *Outcome Indicators for Policy and Systems Change: Controlling High Cholesterol.* Atlanta, GA: Centers for Disease Control and Prevention.

Montz, E., and M. Seshamani. 2009. *A success story in American health care: Community-based prevention in Nebraska.* http://healthreform.gov/reports/success_nebraska/ (accessed December 18, 2009).

4

Interventions Directed at the General Population

This chapter focuses on a number of interventions to address population-based risk factors—overweight, obesity, high sodium intake, low intake of potassium, unhealthy diet, high levels of alcohol consumption, low levels of physical activity—that are known to increase the risk of hypertension in the general population. Some trends in these risk factors, as noted in Chapter 2, are concerning because they are on the rise or have not decreased over time. This chapter includes an examination of the attributable fraction of hypertension due to each risk factor and an estimate of the benefit associated with interventions directed toward reducing these risk factors and their potential effectiveness relative to one another. Estimating the percentage of hypertension cases in a population attributable to different risk factors is useful as part of the process of setting public health priorities. However, these estimates do not apply to individual patients with hypertension, who may each have a different combination of factors contributing to their elevation in blood pressure.

The chapter also discusses community and environmental health determinants of hypertension, and the importance of considering health disparities. Potential interventions such as community and environmental interventions, and public education and media and social marketing campaigns are considered. Finally, the chapter ends with a concluding statement and recommendations.

METHODOLOGY

This section addresses the methodology used in prioritizing modifiable risk factors for intervention. The committee's selection of priority interventions was based primarily on the potential impact on the population if the risk factor were eliminated (population attributable risk). One method to compute population attributable fractions for hypertension is to identify prospective observational studies that have analyzed the association between a given risk factor and the incidence of hypertension. Using the relative risk (RR) between a given risk factor and incident hypertension, as well as the prevalence of that risk factor in the population, the attributable fraction can be computed as follows, where Pe is the prevalence of the exposure in the population:

$$AF = \{ \ (RR-1) \times P_e \ \}f \div \{ \ ([RR-1] \times P_e) + 1 \ \}$$

To compute the attributable fractions for various risk factors, the committee used dichotomized RR estimates and estimates of the prevalence of these risk factors in the population.

Prospective studies pertaining to each of the modifiable risk factors (i.e., overweight and obesity, physical inactivity, heavy alcohol use, high salt intake, low potassium intake, and Western-style diet) were examined. A range of relative risks or odds ratios were extracted from these analyses, and accordingly, a range of attributable fractions for hypertension were computed. In addition, an aggregate relative risk was derived from the available literature, and a corresponding aggregate attributable fraction was computed.

A second method to compute population attributable fractions for hypertension is to identify randomized controlled trials, which report the effect of lifestyle modification interventions on blood pressure. Preferably, large-scale systemic reviews that pool the data from multiple randomized trials could provide a useful aggregate effect estimate (and range of estimates). In order to use these effect estimates to compute attributable fractions, a estimation of the mean blood pressure (and standard deviation) among the exposed population (i.e., the population with the risk factor) must be made, and two assumptions must also then be made: (1) that the blood pressure follows a normal distribution and (2) that applying the intervention to the exposed population would lead to a change in the mean blood pressure of that population that is identical to the pooled estimates reported from meta-analyses. Using a normal distribution function for systolic blood pressure (because most hypertension is systolic hypertension) and computing the percent of exposed individuals with a systolic blood pressure ≥ 140 mm Hg, the change in hypertension prevalence as a result of the intervention can then be estimated as the change in prevalence of hypertension using the normal distribution multiplied by the prevalence of the risk factor in the population. Finally, the attributable fraction of hypertension due to the risk factor can then be computed by dividing the intervention-induced change in hypertension prevalence by the prevalence of hypertension in the whole population. Using this methodology, attributable risks were computed for the viable modifiable risk factors.

The committee also notes that much of the evidence contained in the following sections comes primarily from observational epidemiological investigations, which are mainly cross-sectional or prospective in nature, and randomized intervention trials. Each of these has its strengths and limitations. The observational studies are often large and long term and are thus able to evaluate both the incidence of hypertension and blood pressure as outcomes, but results can be distorted by unmeasured or poorly measured confounding factors. Randomized trials can directly evaluate an intervention, or change in exposure, and reduce the likelihood of confounding, thus providing valuable evidence for causation. However, most of these trials have only evaluated changes in blood pressure rather than incidence of hypertensions because of their limited size and duration. Estimates of attributable risks were generally similar when obtained using the different approaches, which enhances the validity of conclusions.

PROMOTE WEIGHT LOSS AMONG OVERWEIGHT PERSONS

According to data from the National Center for Health Statistics, approximately two-thirds of U.S. adults are overweight or obese (Table 4-1). In the prospective studies that have examined body mass index (BMI) in relation to adjusted risks of incident hypertension, overweight and obesity have been consistently and significantly associated with a higher risk of incident hypertension (Ascherio et al., 1992; Friedman et al., 1988; Gelber et al., 2007; Hu et al., 2004; Huang et al., 1998; Ishikawa-Takata et al., 2002). The most modest association was observed in 17,441 Finnish men and women who were followed for 11 years (Hu et al., 2004). Compared to individuals with a normal BMI, the adjusted relative risk for hypertension among those who were overweight was 1.24 (1.05-1.46) in women and 1.18 (1.01-1.39) in men; among obese individuals, the relative risk of hypertension was 1.32 (1.07-1.62) in women and 1.66 (1.35-2.04) in men. The authors did not provide a summary estimate for a BMI ≥ 25 compared to normal-weight men, but if these relative risks are projected onto the current U.S. population (with roughly equal proportions of overweight—34 percent—and obese—32 percent), then an average relative risk of 1.3 may be a reasonable estimate of the association of overweight and obesity with hypertension among women (and a somewhat stronger association among

TABLE 4-1 Risk Factor: Overweight and Obesity

Modifiable Risk Factor	Definition	Prevalence (source)
Overweight and obesity	BMI ≥25 kg/m^2 Relative risk, mean (range) 1.7 (1.3-2.6)	0.66 (NCHS, 2006) Attributable fraction, mean (range) 32% (17-51%)

Lifestyle intervention	References	Initial SBP[a]	Change in SBP	Anticipated change in HTN[b] prevalence	Attributable fraction
Weight loss	(Horvath et al., 2008) (Ebrahim and Smith, 1998)	135 (18)	−6 (−3 to −10)	8% (4-13%)	28%
			−5 (−2 to −8)	7% (3-10%)	24%

[a] Systolic blood pressure.
[b] Hypertension.

men). The prospective study with the strongest association between BMI and hypertension was the Nurses' Health Study. Nurses who had a BMI of 25.0 to 25.9 had a 2.6-fold (2.3-2.8) increased risk of developing hypertension during the subsequent 16 years compared to the leanest women, and the risk increased stepwise with higher BMIs (Huang et al., 1998). The relative risk estimates for the other prospective studies fell between these values, and the mean relative risk was 1.7. Using this mean and range of effect estimates and a population prevalence of overweight and obesity of 66 percent, it can be estimated that approximately 32 percent (range between 17 and 51 percent) of new hypertension cases occurring in the United States can be attributed to overweight and obesity (Table 4-1).

Important supportive evidence for these epidemiological findings has been provided by a series of randomized trials that have analyzed the effect of weight loss interventions on blood pressure; the majority of these studies succeeded in reducing weight in the intervention group by about 5 kg (Anderssen et al., 1995; Croft et al., 1986; Jalkanen, 1991; Stevens et al., 2001; The Trials of Hypertension Prevention Collaborative Research Group, 1992, 1997; Wassertheil-Smoller et al., 1992). Two meta-analyses have been performed that pool the results of these trials. The more recent meta-analysis, by Horvath et al. (2008), demonstrated a 6 mm Hg (−3 to −10 mm Hg) decrease in systolic blood pressure with weight loss. The older study by Ebrahim and Smith (1998) found a 5 mm Hg (−2 to −8 mm Hg) fall in systolic blood pressure with weight loss Based on these results, an intervention (to reduce weight by about 5 kg, or 10 lbs) applied to overweight and obese members of the population would hypothetically reduce the overall population prevalence of hypertension by 7 to 8 percent. Additionally, an estimated 24-28 percent of hypertension in the United States may be attributable to overweight and obesity, an estimate that is consistent with the attributable fractions computed using observational data.

DECREASE SODIUM INTAKE

Based upon 2004 statistics using calculated intakes of sodium, 87 percent of U.S. adults consumed what is considered excess sodium based on the Dietary Guidelines for Americans (>100 mmol of sodium ≅ >2,400 mg sodium ≅ >6,000 mg of salt [sodium chloride]) (NCHS, 2008) (Table 4-2).[1] Further, the Dietary Guidelines for Americans, 2005, and the American

---

[1] Conversion factors: In view of the variability of the published data referred to in this report the following conversion information is provided. To convert millimoles (mmol) to milligrams (mg) of sodium, chloride, or sodium chloride, multiply mmol by 23, 35.5, or 58.5 (the respective molecular weights of sodium, chloride, and sodium chloride), respectively. To convert millimoles (mmol) of potassium to mg of potassium, multiply by 39, the molecular weight of potassium.

TABLE 4-2 Risk Factor: High Salt Intake

Modifiable Risk Factor	Definition	Prevalence (source)
High salt intake	≥2,400 mg/day sodium **Relative risk, mean (range)** 1.3 (1.2-1.4)	0.87 (HHS, 2008) **Attributable fraction, mean (range)** 32% (17-51%)

Lifestyle intervention	References	Initial SBP[a]	Change in SBP	Anticipated change in HTN[b] prevalence	Attributable fraction
Reduce salt intake	(He and MacGregor, 2004)	131 (19)	−4 (−3 to −5)	6% (5-8%)	21%

[a] Systolic blood pressure.
[b] Hypertension.

Heart Association recommend that African Americans and persons who are middle aged or older or who have hypertension should consume less than 1,500 mg of sodium daily; with this added criterion the number consuming excess sodium is substantially higher than 87 percent (AHA, 2009; HHS and USDA, 2005). However, calculated sodium intake may not be accurate because the large majority of sodium in the U.S. food supply is added in the processing and manufacturing of foods and a large and increasing amount is used in the fast food industry. The amounts added can vary widely by brand and with time, making calculations difficult, and the smaller amounts added at home can also be challenging to quantify. Unfortunately, 24-hour urinary sodium excretion, which provides the best measure of sodium intake, has never been assessed in a nationally representative sample of the U.S. population, so that the true distribution of intakes in the United States is not known.

Very few prospective studies have addressed the association between antecedent dietary salt intake and the risk of developing hypertension. This is probably due mainly to the difficulty in accurately ascertaining sodium intake in large cohorts because most sodium is added in the manufacturing and processing of food rather than being intrinsic to food itself. As mentioned by the authors, misclassification of sodium intake potentially explains the absence of an association between estimated sodium intake and hypertension in the Nurses' Health Study and the Health Professionals Follow-up Study (Ascherio et al., 1992, 1996). In cross-sectional observational studies, positive associations have been seen between sodium intake (as assessed by 24-hour urine collections) and blood pressure or prevalent hypertension (Karppanen and Mervaala, 2006; Stamler, 1997).

Numerous interventional studies of salt intake and blood pressure (analyzed as a continuous variable) of various quality and duration have been performed. Some of these sodium reduction trials had sufficiently long periods of follow-up to ascertain hypertension as a secondary end point (Goldstein, 1990; The Trials of Hypertension Prevention Collaborative Research Group, 1992, 1997). The Hypertension Prevention Trial randomized men and women ages 25-49 years to one of five counseling groups, including no counseling, counseling to reduce sodium, counseling to reduce sodium and increase potassium, counseling to reduce sodium and calories, and counseling to reduce calories. After 3 years of follow-up, sodium intake was reduced 10 percent (34 mmol per day), and the odds ratio for incident hypertension among the no-counseling group compared to the low-sodium group was 1.4. Phase I of The Trials of Hypertension Prevention (TOHP-I) enrolled more than 2,000 men and women ages 30 to 54 years with diastolic blood pressures of 80 to 89 mm Hg and randomized them to one of four groups: control (no intervention), low sodium, weight loss, and stress reduction (The Trials of Hypertension Prevention Collaborative Research

Group, 1992). Participants were followed for 18 months. Compared to the control, the sodium intervention led to a reduction in sodium intake of 44 mmol per day; the odds ratio for incident hypertension among controls was 1.3 (The Trials of Hypertension Prevention Collaborative Research Group, 1992). Phase II (TOHP-II) randomized more than 2,000 overweight men and women ages 30 to 54 years with diastolic blood pressures of 83-89 mm Hg and systolic blood pressures <140 mm Hg to usual care, counseling to achieve an 80-mmol-per-day (2 grams) sodium diet, weight loss, or a combination of weight loss and low-sodium diet (The Trials of Hypertension Prevention Collaborative Research Group, 1997). Counseling on sodium restriction led to a 40-mmol-per-day reduction in sodium intake. Through four years of follow-up, the odds ratio of incident hypertension among the control group compared to the sodium restriction group was 1.2 (The Trials of Hypertension Prevention Collaborative Research Group, 1997). While other randomized trials that included sodium restriction as one intervention also had extended follow-up and ascertainment of hypertension incidence (e.g., the Primary Prevention Trial and the PREMIER clinical trial of comprehensive lifestyle modification for blood pressure control; (Elmer et al., 2006; Stamler et al., 1989), sodium restriction was examined in combination with other factors rather than in isolation. Using this range of effect estimates and a population prevalence of 87 percent for high salt intake, it can be estimated that between 15 and 26 percent of new hypertension cases occurring in the United States could be attributed to a high salt intake with an average estimate from the available studies of 21 percent.

The most up-to-date systematic reviews of blood pressure-lowering trials via sodium restriction were published by He and MacGregor (2004) and Dickinson et al. (2006); both studies reported essentially identical pooled estimates. He and MacGregor (2004) analyzed 31 trials of at least one-month duration in which the sodium intake (measured by sodium excreted in 24-hour urine) in the treatment group was reduced by at least 40 mmol (approximately 1,000 mg of sodium, or 2,300 mg of salt-sodium chloride). The average sodium reduction in these studies was 76 mmol (about 1,750 mg of sodium, or 4,438 mg of salt); this represents less than half the daily salt intake (9-12 grams) of average Americans (He and MacGregor, 2004). The pooled estimate for systolic blood pressure reduction from sodium restriction was 4 mm Hg (−3 to −5 mm Hg). By using these estimates and a prevalence of sodium excess in the general population of 0.87, the prevalence of hypertension could potentially be reduced by 5 to 8 percent if all Americans consuming a high-salt diet lowered their salt intake by about 4.5 grams per day. The corresponding attributable fraction of hypertension due to sodium excess is approximately 21 percent, precisely what was found when data from intervention studies with hypertension as the dichotomous outcome were analyzed.

INCREASE POTASSIUM AND INTAKE OF
FRUITS AND VEGETABLES

Of all of the modifiable risk factors for hypertension, one of the most prevalent is an inadequate consumption of potassium based on the current Dietary Reference Intake (DRI) criteria (IOM, 2005). In a recent report from the CDC (NCHS, 2008), approximately 2 percent of U.S. adults met the current guidelines for dietary potassium intake (≥4.7 grams per day, or 4,700 mg), but insufficient potassium intake is most prevalent among blacks and Hispanics, among whom the proportion consuming an adequate amount of potassium was close to zero percent. Of note, the primary basis for the DRI of 4.7 grams per day for potassium is its beneficial effect on blood pressure and stroke (IOM, 2005). Specifically, this amount of potassium, provided as a supplement, was needed to counteract the effect of a high salt load among 10 black men; among white men, 2.7 grams per day appeared to be adequate. In the 2005 U.S. Dietary Guidelines, the value of 4.7 grams per day based on supplemental potassium was translated into recommendations for high consumption of fruits, vegetables, and dairy products, which are major sources of this nutrient (HHS and USDA, 2005) (Table 4-3).

Observational studies that have examined the association between potassium intake and incident hypertension are conflicting (Ascherio et al., 1992, 1996; Chien et al., 2008; Dyer et al., 1994; Lever et al., 1981). While some cross-sectional analyses of 24-hour urinary potassium excretion and blood pressure have demonstrated an inverse association (Dyer et al., 1994; Lever et al., 1981), prospective studies have not shown clear associations. In both the large-scale Nurses' Health Study and the Health Professionals Follow-up Study, higher intakes of potassium ascertained from repeated food-frequency questionnaires were inversely associated with risk of hypertension, but it was difficult to determine the independence from other dietary factors in multivariate analyses (Ascherio et al., 1992, 1996). In a recent study among 1,523 men and women in Taiwan, the incidence of hypertension was ascertained during eight years of follow-up after a baseline 24-hour urine collection; the relative risk comparing the highest to lowest quartile of potassium excretion was 0.98 (0.78-1.23) after multivariate adjustment (Chien et al., 2008). Whether a single measure of urinary potassium is adequate for characterizing long-term potassium intake in this population is unclear.

Numerous randomized trials have examined whether potassium supplementation lowers blood pressure, and the overall evidence indicates a benefit although this has not been seen in all studies (Appel et al., 2006). Four meta-analyses have been published that have pooled these studies (Cappuccio and MacGregor, 1991; Dickinson et al., 2006; Geleijnse et

TABLE 4-3 Risk Factor: Low Potassium Intake

Modifiable Risk Factor		Definition		Prevalence (source)	
Low potassium intake		<4,700 mg/day potassium		0.98 (Sondik, 2008)	
Lifestyle intervention	References	Initial SBP[a]	Change in SBP	Anticipated change in HTN[b] prevalence	Attributable fraction
Increase potassium intake	(Whelton et al., 1997)	131 (19)	−3 (−2 to −4)	5% (4-7%)	17%

[a] Systolic blood pressure.
[b] Hypertension.

al., 2003; Whelton et al., 1997). Three studies found significant pooled blood pressure reductions with potassium supplementation (Cappuccio and MacGregor, 1991; Geleijnse et al., 2003; Whelton et al., 1997), while the most recent (which excluded trials of very short duration, those that included children and pregnant women, and those that included participants on blood pressure medications that were altered during the study period) did not detect a significant effect (Dickinson et al., 2006). Nevertheless, the pooled estimate from that meta-analysis suggested a favorable effect of potassium (a 3.9 mm Hg decrease in blood pressure), despite the insignificant p-value (Dickinson et al., 2006). In the most comprehensive of these meta-analyses, Whelton et al. synthesized 33 randomized trials of potassium supplementation and reported a pooled reduction of systolic blood pressure by 3 mm Hg (–2 to –4 mm Hg), and a pooled reduction in diastolic blood pressure of 2 mm Hg (–1 to –4 mm Hg) (Whelton et al., 1997).

Although recommendations for high intakes of fruits and vegetables in the U.S. Dietary Guidelines are based largely on studies of potassium supplementation and blood pressure, the effect of increasing fruits and vegetables on blood pressure was investigated directly in the Dietary Approaches to Stop Hypertension (DASH) study (Appel et al., 1997). In this study, one intervention group was fed 8.5 servings of fruits and vegetables (analyzed potassium intake 4,101 mg per day), whereas the comparison group received 3.6 servings per day (analyzed potassium intake 1,752 mg per day). The fruits-and-vegetables diet reduced systolic blood pressure by 2.8 mm Hg more (p < 0.001) and diastolic blood pressure by 1.1 mm Hg more than the control diet (p = 0.07), which is consistent with the potassium content of these foods. DASH results showing reduced systolic and diastolic blood pressure with an increase in dietary fruit and vegetables have also been reported by researchers in the United Kingdom (John et al., 2002).

Using the results of the meta-analysis of Whelton and colleagues in which the dose of potassium supplementation was typically 60 mmol per day, and the assumption that the entire population could increase its intake to 4,700 mg per day, the prevalence of hypertension could hypothetically be reduced by 4 to 7 percent. Further, the attributable fraction corresponding to insufficient potassium intake is approximately 17 percent.

There is evidence that increasing the potassium intake of the general U.S. population would have favorable effects on blood pressure, but the methods of doing this need to be considered. The high intake of fruits and vegetables in the DASH study (8.5 servings per day) is a desirable goal, but increases to this level will be difficult to achieve in the medium-term future because there has been little increase in these foods in the United States (if french-fried potatoes are not included) despite strong encouragement to do so. Whether smaller increases would have similar benefits is not clear. Potassium supplements for the general population are not usually advised because of possible adverse gastrointestinal effects (Cohn et al., 2000) and concern about the development of hyperkalemia among individuals with chronic renal failure or on potassium-sparing diuretics. However, maintenance of normal potassium homeostasis typically does not become problematic in people with kidney disease until the glomerular filtration rate falls below 20 mL/min. This severity of kidney disease is uncommon in the general population (about 0.1 percent of the population), and awareness is higher among these individuals (Coresh et al., 2005). Another strategy to increase potassium intake is by the use of "modified salt" in food preparation in which part of the sodium chloride is replaced by potassium chloride. This has the double advantage of decreasing sodium and increasing potassium intake, and the likelihood of excessive potassium intake is limited by its effect on flavor. The more widespread use of these substitutes, accompanied by clear labeling for those whose intake of potassium should be limited for medical reasons, deserves further consideration.

CONSUME A HEALTHY DIET

In many studies of vegetarians and rural populations of developing countries, the eating patterns of these groups have been associated with lower blood pressure and lower rates of hypertension (Armstrong et al., 1977; Cruz-Coke et al., 1964; He et al., 1991; Klag et al., 1995; Poulter et al., 1985, 1990; Sacks and Kass, 1988; Sacks et al., 1974; Sever et al., 1980). For example, among young men and women living in the Boston area, the prevalence of hypertension was approximately 20 percent among nonvegetarians vs. zero percent among vegetarians (Sacks and Kass, 1988). In a study of South African blacks, the odds ratio for prevalent hypertension comparing urban vs. tribal dwelling Xhosa and Zulu people was 2.1, although this was unadjusted. When comparing migrants from a rural to an urban area of China with those who had not migrated, the adjusted odds ratio for prevalent hypertension was 1.91 (standardized for slightly different odds ratios in men and women) (He et al., 1991). These observations led to the hypothesis that interventions involving a healthy overall eating pattern might be more clearly related to lower blood pressure than those focused on single nutrients. This led investigators of the DASH trial to propose a healthy eating plan that would lower blood pressure (Appel et al., 2006). This diet was high in fruits, vegetables, and low-fat dairy products and low in saturated fat and sweets (Appel et al., 1997), and was thus high in potassium, calcium, magnesium, and fiber.

Published data from observational studies that provide an estimate of the association between an overall healthy diet or the DASH dietary pattern and incident hypertension are generally limited. Investigators at the

European Investigation into Cancer and Nutrition (EPIC)-Potsdam Study did analyze the association between a DASH dietary pattern and incident hypertension, but among the population with sufficient dietary data, only 123 incident hypertension cases occurred; a DASH-style diet was inversely associated with hypertension, but this was not statistically significant (Schulze et al., 2003). The one prospective study that did find a significant association between a DASH-style diet and incident hypertension was the Nurses' Health Study II (Forman et al., 2009). Among more than 83,000 women followed for 14 years, those in the lowest compared to the highest quintile of DASH score (a score generated from factor analysis to reflect a DASH eating style) had a 1.22-fold increased risk of incident hypertension (1.15-1.30) after adjustment for multiple factors (Forman et al., 2009).

The DASH trial itself had insufficiently long-term follow-up to demonstrate a persistent change in blood pressure at one year, or a change in hypertension incidence (Ard et al., 2004), despite providing clear evidence that the DASH diet lowers blood pressure. Although the PREMIER trial analyzed incident hypertension at 18 months of follow-up, the DASH diet was not analyzed in isolation (Elmer et al., 2006). Rather, the DASH diet was combined with weight loss, sodium restriction, and physical activity. Compared to the group receiving weight loss, sodium restriction, and physical activity without the DASH eating plan, the addition of the DASH eating plan was associated with a relative risk for incident hypertension of 0.93 (0.75-1.15) (Elmer et al., 2006). By using the range of effect estimates from comparisons of populations and cohort studies and a conservative estimate of the population prevalence of a Western-style diet of 75 percent (it is probably higher), it can be estimated that between 13 and 40 percent of new hypertension cases occurring in the United States can be attributed to a Western-style diet, with an aggregate estimate from the few available studies of 31 percent (Table 4-4).

There are no meta-analyses of dietary pattern interventions and blood pressure lowering. Therefore, the attributable fraction of hypertension as a consequence of a Western-style diet was computed from the DASH randomized trial, in which the combination (DASH) diet lowered blood pressure by approximately 6 mm Hg (-4 to -7 mm Hg) (Appel et al., 1997). The reduction in blood pressure on the DASH diet was greater than in a parallel intervention that only increased fruit and vegetable consumption; however, the DASH diet also contained more fruits and vegetables, thus complicating the conclusions. The DASH-sodium trial is not included in this estimation because dietary pattern change was not the sole intervention (Sacks et al., 2001). Again, by assuming a prevalence of a Western-style diet in the United States of 0.75, a DASH diet intervention targeted to all adults who ate this type of diet could potentially reduce the prevalence of hypertension in the population by 6 to 10 percent. The estimated attributable fraction

TABLE 4-4 Risk Factor: Western-Style (Unhealthy) Diet

Modifiable Risk Factor		Definition		Prevalence (source)
Western-style diet		A diet emphasizing red and processed meats, refined grains, fats, and sweetened foods		0.75 (conservative estimate)
		Relative risk, mean (range) 1.6 (1.2-1.9)		**Attributable fraction, mean (range)** 31% (13-40%)
Lifestyle intervention	References	Initial SBP[a]	Change in SBP	Anticipated change in HTN[b] prevalence	Attributable fraction
DASH eating plan	(Appel et al., 1997)	131 (11)	−6 (−4 to −7)	8% (6-10%)	28%

[a] Systolic blood pressure.
[b] Hypertension.

of hypertension prevalence due to a Western-style diet is consequently 28 percent.

Subsequent to the initial DASH study, two important enhancements have been documented. The first is salt reduction, discussed later under "Multiple Dietary Interventions," which led to an additional decrease in blood pressure. The second is partial replacement (10 percent of energy) of the high amount of carbohydrate in the DASH diet with either unsaturated fat or protein, which was addressed in the OmniHeart study (Appel et al., 2005). Both substitutions significantly reduced systolic blood pressure (by 1.3 to 1.4 mm Hg overall and by about 3 mm among those with hypertension) and also improved blood lipids. The finding that replacement of carbohydrate by either unsaturated fat or protein reduces blood pressure suggests a role of carbohydrate reduction rather than increased intake of protein or unsaturated fat in control of hypertension.

The initial DASH diet has an important benefit in reducing blood pressure, but the OmniHeart study showed that further reduction in blood pressure is possible if the high carbohydrate content of the DASH diet is reduced by partial replacement with either protein or unsaturated fat and that blood lipids are also improved. These findings are consistent with many controlled feeding studies that show improvements in blood lipids when carbohydrate is replaced with unsaturated fats (Mensink et al., 2003). Also, in the Nurses' Health Study a dietary pattern lower in carbohydrates and higher in unsaturated fats and vegetable sources of protein was associated with lower risk of coronary heart disease and type 2 diabetes (Halton et al., 2006, 2008). The high consumption of dairy products in the DASH diet is of concern because many studies have found this to be associated with fatal prostate cancer, particularly the aggressive form, and a recent review concluded that high consumption of dairy products probably increases the risk of prostate cancer (World Cancer Research Fund, 2007). Thus, an overall diet for good health would probably include lower amounts of carbohydrate and dairy products than the original DASH diet.

REDUCE EXCESSIVE ALCOHOL INTAKE

According to 2001-2007 government data, the prevalence of heavy drinking (defined as ≥3 drinks per day in men and ≥2 drinks per day in women) among U.S. adults is 5 percent (CDC, 2008a) (Table 4-5). At least nine prospective cohort studies have examined the independent association between alcohol consumption and the risk of hypertension (Ascherio et al., 1992; Friedman et al., 1988; Fuchs et al., 2001; Lorenzo et al., 2002; Ohmori et al., 2002; Sesso et al., 2008; Stranges et al., 2004; Thadhani et al., 2002; Witteman et al., 1990). Although they varied in the way in which alcohol intake was classified and not all examined the association using cur-

TABLE 4-5 Risk Factor: Heavy Alcohol Intake

Modifiable Risk Factor	Definition	Prevalence (source)
Heavy alcohol intake	Mean of ≥3 (in men) or ≥2 (in women) alcoholic beverages per day **Relative risk, mean (range)** 1.7 (1.2-2.3)	0.05 (CDC, 2008b) **Attributable fraction, mean (range)** 3% (1-6%)

Lifestyle intervention	References	Initial SBP[a]	Change in SBP	Anticipated change in HTN[b] prevalence	Attributable fraction
Reduce alcohol intake	(Xin et al., 2001)	132 (18)	−3 (−2 to −4)	0.3% (0.2-0.4%)	1%

[a] Systolic blood pressure.
[b] Hypertension.

rently recommended thresholds of ≥3 alcoholic beverages per day for men and ≥2 alcoholic beverages per day for women (on average), they provide useful information in determining the attributable risk of alcohol use for hypertension. The lowest relative risk was observed among white men in the Atherosclerosis Risk in Communities (ARIC) Study who consumed 3 or more alcoholic beverages per day (RR = 1.2 [0.85-1.67]) (Fuchs et al., 2001). The same study also reported the strongest association (RR = 2.3 [1.11-4.86]) among black men who drank 3 or more alcoholic beverages per day. The other eight studies reported risk estimates that fell between 1.2 and 2.3. The average relative risk of hypertension for those drinking alcohol in excess from all nine cohorts was 1.7. Supportive evidence regarding the potential benefit of interventions to reduce alcohol use comes from a systematic review of 15 randomized controlled trials of alcohol reduction in heavy drinkers that demonstrated a significant pooled reduction in blood pressure (Xin et al., 2001). Given the consistency of observational and interventional evidence, a program to reduce alcohol consumption among adults drinking excessive amounts is a viable option to reduce the prevalence of hypertension. However, based upon a relative risk of 1.7 and a prevalence of heavy alcohol use of 5 percent, the estimated fraction of hypertension attributable to excess alcohol use is low: 3 percent (range, 1-6 percent) (Forman, 2009).

One meta-analysis pooled results from 14 randomized trials of alcohol reduction among heavy drinkers, with 13 of the 14 studies having a follow-up of at least one month (Xin et al., 2001). The authors reported that alcohol restriction resulted in a pooled reduction of systolic blood pressure of 3 mm Hg (–2 to –4 mm Hg). Using these figures in conjunction with the prevalence of excess alcohol intake, an alcohol restriction program applied in all population members who drink alcohol to excess (i.e., ≥2 drinks per day in women and ≥3 drinks per day in men) may reduce the overall population prevalence of hypertension by 0.2 to 0.4 percent. The estimated attributable fraction of hypertension due to alcohol excess using this method (1 percent) is consistent with the estimates derived from observational studies.

INCREASE PHYSICAL ACTIVITY

Approximately 69 percent of the U.S. adult population in 2001 did not meet the CDC guidelines for leisure time physical activity of 5 days per week of moderate-intensity exercise or 3 days per week of vigorous exercise (CDC, 2003). Several large, prospective, cohort studies have examined the association between physical activity and incident hypertension, although none has categorized physical activity according to current guidelines for moderate or vigorous physical activity (Graham et al., 2007; Hayashi et al.,

1999; Hu et al., 2004; Parker et al., 2007; Pereira et al., 1999). Although most of these studies supported an inverse relation between physical activity and risk of hypertension, the ARIC study reported an inverse association only among white men. The lack of apparent benefit in other demographic groups may have been due to their lower levels of recreational activity (Pereira et al., 1999). However, the Coronary Artery Risk Development in Young Adults (CARDIA) study found that increased levels of physical activity reduced the risk of incident hypertension, and the association remained constant after adjusting for race, gender, and other variables (Parker et al., 2007). The most impressive association was present among Finnish men, in whom a lack of moderate or vigorous regular physical activity was associated with a 64 percent increase in the risk of developing hypertension (Hu et al., 2004). Other cohort studies reported more modest, although significant, inverse associations. The mean relative risk estimate from these cohort studies is 1.3. Using this estimate and a population prevalence of 69 percent for lack of regular exercise, it can be estimated that 17 percent of new hypertension cases (range 0 to 29 percent) occurring in the United States can be attributed to lack of regular exercise (Table 4-6).

Two large scale meta-analyses have analyzed randomized trials of exercise interventions and reduction in blood pressure (Kelley and Sharpe Kelley, 2001; Whelton et al., 2002). The more recent, by Whelton and colleagues, reported that exercise led to a 4 mm Hg (–3 to –5 mm Hg) reduction in systolic blood pressure. The older study by Kelley and Sharpe Kelley (2001) documented a more modest reduction by 2 mm Hg (–1 to –4 mm Hg) (Kelley and Sharpe Kelley, 2001; Whelton et al., 2002). The meta-analysis published by Dickinson et al. (2006) examining multiple lifestyle interventions found a pooled effect for exercise similar to that found by Whelton et al. (2002). As with overweight and obesity, the anticipated change in hypertension prevalence and the attributable fraction can be estimated from these values using similar techniques. Implementation of an exercise program among members of the population who are physically inactive would hypothetically reduce the overall prevalence of hypertension by 4 to 6 percent. Furthermore, the fraction of hypertension attributable to physical inactivity is estimated by this method to be 14-21 percent, consistent with estimates using observational data.

MULTIPLE DIETARY INTERVENTIONS

Several high-quality randomized trials have investigated the effects of multiple risk factor reduction on blood pressure. The DASH-sodium trial was a 2 × 2 factorial trial that randomized participants to either a Western-style diet or the DASH diet and to one of three levels of sodium intake (150 mmol, 100 mmol, and 50 mmol) (Sacks et al., 2001). The achieved

TABLE 4-6 Risk Factors: Physical Inactivity

Modifiable Risk Factor	Definition	Prevalence (source)
Physical inactivity	No sessions of light/moderate or vigorous physical activity lasting ≥10 minutes	0.69 (NHIS 2006 survey) (NCHS, 2003)
	Relative risk, mean (range)	**Attributable fraction, mean (range)**
	1.3 (1.0-1.6)	17% (0-29%)

Lifestyle intervention	References	Initial SBP[a]	Change in SBP	Anticipated change in HTN[b] prevalence	Attributable fraction
Increase physical activity	(Whelton et al., 2002)	131 (17)	−4 (−3 to −5)	6% (4-7%)	21%
	(Kelley and Sharpe Kelley, 2001)		−2 (−1 to −4)	4% (1-6%)	14%

[a] Systolic blood pressure.
[b] Hypertension.

sodium intakes were similar to these targeted intakes, and the highest- vs. lowest-sodium groups were separated by 77 mmol per day. Comparing the Western-style, high-sodium diet with the DASH lowest-sodium diet, the reduction in systolic blood pressure was approximately 9 mm Hg (–4 to –14 mm Hg). If U.S. adults on a Western-style, high-salt diet were fed a DASH-style, low-salt diet, hypertension prevalence might be reduced by 14 to 22 percent (Table 4-7). The corresponding attributable fraction of hypertension due to a Western-style, high-salt diet is estimated to be 59 percent.

The second trial of multiple risk factor reduction was the PREMIER trial, which randomized participants either to usual counseling; to a behavioral intervention targeted to reduce sodium intake, reduce weight, and improve physical conditioning; or to a behavioral intervention that combined these interventions with the DASH diet (Elmer et al., 2006). The PREMIER trial, unlike DASH-sodium, was not a feeding trial, and as a consequence the separation between the groups was not as dramatic; this has been seen in most lifestyle intervention studies conducted in environments that are generally not supportive of healthy behaviors. For example, the sodium intake at 18 months of follow-up was 168 mmol per day (nearly 10 grams of salt) in the control group and 153 mmol (nearly 9 grams of salt) in the targeted multiple intervention groups (Elmer et al., 2006). Both of these sodium intake levels would be considered sodium excess. At 18 months, systolic blood pressure was reduced by 2 mm Hg (0 to –4 mm Hg).

The overall potential for reduction of hypertension by dietary factors, weight control, and regular physical activity has not been addressed directly. The attributable risks shown for individual factors in Table 4-8 cannot simply be added because this would not take into account their interactions, and for this reason the sum can be more than 100 percent. However, if the 59 percent of risk attributable to the DASH diet with sodium reduction is taken as a base, to which reduction in carbohydrate, weight loss, and increased physical activity could be added, it can be appreciated qualitatively that a very large majority of hypertension is potentially preventable.

OTHER POTENTIAL INTERVENTIONS

The committee considered other interventions that have been hypothesized to reduce blood pressure including increasing intakes of calcium, magnesium, folic acid, fiber, fish oil, and vitamin D and reducing stress and use of analgesics. For each, the evidence was considered to be inadequate to consider as a priority area of intervention.

TABLE 4-7 Risk Factors: Multiple Interventions

Lifestyle intervention	References	Initial SBP[a]	Change in SBP	Anticipated change in HTN[b] prevalence	Attributable fraction
	(Sacks et al., 2001)	134 (10)	-9 (-4 to -14)	17% (14-22%)	59%
	(Elmer et al., 2006)	135 (10)	-2 (0 to -4)	6% (0-11%)	21%

[a] Systolic blood pressure.
[b] Hypertension.

TABLE 4-8 Modifiable Risk Factors and Attributable Fractions Based on Interventional Studies

Lifestyle intervention	References	Initial SBP[a]	Change in SBP	Anticipated change in HTN[b] prevalence	Attributable fraction
Weight loss	(Horvath et al., 2008)	135 (18)	-6 (-3 to -10)	8% (4-13%)	28%
	(Ebrahim, 1998)		-5 (-2 to -8)	7% (3-10%)	24%
Reduce salt intake	(He and MacGregor, 2004)	131 (19)	-4 (-3 to -5)	6% (5-8%)	21%
DASH eating plan (healthy eating)	(Appel et al., 1997)	131 (11)	-6 (-4 to -7)	8% (6-10%)	28%
Increase potassium intake	(Whelton et al., 1997)	131 (19)	-3 (-2 to -4)	5% (4-7%)	17%
Increase physical activity	(Kelley and Sharpe Kelley, 2001)	131 (17)	-4 (-3 to -5)	6% (4-7%)	21%
	(Whelton et al., 2002)		-2 (-1 to -4)	4% (1-6%)	14%
Reduce alcohol intake	(Xin et al., 2001)	132 (18)	-3 (-2 to -4)	0.3% (0.2-0.4%)	1%

[a] Systolic blood pressure.
[b] Hypertension.

COMMUNITY AND ENVIRONMENTAL INTERVENTIONS

Public health policies that make it easier for Americans to engage in regular, physical activity (leisure time and transportation) and reduce exposure to foods containing high levels of sodium while increasing exposure to foods containing appropriately high levels of potassium are likely to be the most effective means to lower the mean blood pressure of the U.S. population as a whole (Rose, 1992). Thus, approaches to shift the population distribution of blood pressure through the behavioral strategies described above will require addressing community and environmental factors that may limit the ability of individuals to make healthy behavioral choices in the communities where they live and work.

A growing body of work has examined features of neighborhood built environments such as land use patterns, density, and access to destinations; street connectivity and transportation systems; features of urban design; and access to healthy foods and recreational resources in relation to the behaviors of diet and physical activity and related health outcomes of obesity, diabetes, and hypertension. Observational studies have generally concluded that greater population density, land use mix, proximity of nonresidential destinations, pedestrian infrastructure, aesthetics, and safety are linked to more walking (Saelens and Handy, 2008). There is also observational evidence that the presence of resources for physical activity in parks and recreational facilities relates to residents' physical activity levels (Kaczynski and Henderson, 2008). A growing body of work has linked access to healthy foods (as proxied by the presence of supermarkets or other measures of availability) to better diets (Franco et al., 2009; Larson et al., 2009; Moore et al., 2008). Recent work has also shown that neighborhood physical activity and food environments are related to levels and changes over time in obesity, hypertension, and diabetes (Black and Macinko, 2008; Larson et al., 2009; Mujahid et al., 2008a; Papas et al., 2007; Sturm and Datar, 2005, 2008).

Although existing evidence remains limited due to its observational nature, there is growing consensus that efforts to improve population levels of physical activity, diet, and related conditions will have to encompass interventions that address the environments that promote and sustain healthy behaviors (IOM, 2009a). For example, it has been argued that public health efforts to improve physical activity should include design and land use policies that support physical activity, as well as creating and/or increasing access to places for physical activity (Heath et al., 2006; Kahn et al., 2002). Similarly, public health efforts to improve diet will need to address the limited access to healthy foods that has been documented in many communities (Franco et al., 2008; Moore and Diez Roux, 2006; Morland et al.,

2002). Rigorous evaluation of efforts to improve physical activity and food environments will be necessary to guide future action.

Public Education and Media and Social Marketing Campaigns

Public education is an important component of many public health intervention activities. Public education campaigns use a variety of methods and tools—from the dissemination of printed educational materials to very sophisticated, targeted social marketing techniques. Public education campaigns generally strive to raise awareness and disseminate messages, while social marketing techniques focus on changing behaviors. This section discusses the impact of the National High Blood Pressure Education Program and the results of local efforts associated with the Pawtucket Heart Health Program, Minnesota Heart Health Program, and Stanford Five City Project, which were funded by the National Heart, Lung, and Blood Institute (NHLBI) between 1978 and 1980 and included public education efforts to reduce risk factors associated with cardiovascular disease. The section also reviews the VERB™ campaign that targeted physical activity as an example of a successful public education campaign.

National High Blood Pressure Education Program

The National High Blood Pressure Education Program (NHBPEP) was initiated in 1972 and is coordinated by the NHLBI of the National Institutes of Health. The program engages the efforts of federal agencies, professional and voluntary health organizations, state health departments, and community groups to "reduce death and disability related to high blood pressure through programs of professional, patient, and public education." The NHBPEP utilizes strategic partnerships and the development and dissemination of educational materials and programs to work toward achieving the Healthy People 2010 heart disease and stroke objectives. The coordinating committee is engaged in examining critical issues, promoting national activities, and fostering collaboration between organizations, as well as identifying national priorities for the NHBPEP. The mass media efforts directed by the NHBPEP employ the use of fact sheets, brochures, planning kits, posters, print ads, and radio messages to promote professional, patient, and public education. The program also publishes the *Report of the Joint National Committee on Detection, Evaluation, and Treatment of High Blood Pressure*, which provides current guidelines and recommendations for clinicians and community organizations and is widely distributed to state health departments, primary care clinicians, and hypertension control programs. The most recent version of the report was published in 2003, and its update will be released in summer of 2010. The issues and scope identified on the NHBPEP website include the following:

- Excessive stroke mortality in the southeastern United States
- Effective treatment practices
- Utility of lowering the systolic blood pressure in older Americans
- Role of lifestyle changes in preventing and treating hypertension
- Population-based strategies for primary prevention of high blood pressure
- Issues regarding special populations and situations (e.g., African Americans, renal disease, women, children, adolescents)
- Educational strategies directed at professional, patient, and public audiences and community organizations
- Development and support of HEDIS (Healthcare Effectiveness Data and Information Set) hypertension measures.

The NHBPEP measures its progress against the National Health and Nutrition Examination Survey (NHANES) trends in hypertension aware- ness, treatment, and control, as well as the progress made toward the Healthy People 2010 goals. At the program's outset, less than one-quarter of Americans were aware of the relationship between hypertension and stroke and hypertension and heart disease. Hypertension awareness has increased to three-quarters of the population, and three-quarters of Ameri- cans have their blood pressure measured every six months. In 1972, only 16 percent of hypertensive individuals had blood pressure at or below 160/95 mm Hg (the goal at that time). Recent data show that 64 percent would meet the old goal of 160/95 mm Hg, and 29 percent would meet the current goal of 140/90 mm Hg (Jones and Hall, 2002). Hypertension has become a leading reason for physician visits among adults. There has been a 59.6 percent decline in age-adjusted mortality for stroke in the total population since the program's inception and a 55.6 percent decline in coronary heart disease.

Pawtucket Heart Health Program

The Pawtucket Heart Health Program (PHHP) was a community- based research and demonstration project that took place in Pawtucket, Rhode Island, between 1981 and 1993. The program utilized a mass media campaign as well as screening and counseling, grocery store shelf label- ing, and educational programs offered in schools and libraries. It focused on modifying major risk factors for cardiovascular disease including high blood cholesterol levels, high blood pressure, smoking, sedentary lifestyle, and obesity. Random-sample, cross-sectional surveys were administered to residents of Pawtucket and residents of a comparison community who were between the ages of 18 and 64. The resulting analysis showed small, statistically insignificant reductions in blood cholesterol and blood pressure in the Pawtucket community. The projected cardiovascular disease rates were 16 percent lower in Pawtucket during the education program, but fell to 8 percent in the post-intervention period. A study by Carleton et al. (1995) concluded that "[a]ccelerating risk factor changes will likely require a sustained community effort with reinforcement from state, regional, and national policies and programs" (p. 777).

Minnesota Heart Health Program

The Minnesota Heart Health Program took place between 1980 and 1989 and included approximately 400,000 persons in six communities (three intervention and three comparison communities). The program utilized mass and personalized media; adult, youth, and professional education; and community-based health promotion activities. The intervention communities experienced a modest but statistically insignificant decline in measures of systolic and diastolic blood pressure. Baseline and follow-up surveys demonstrated that "[m]any intervention components proved effective in targeted groups. However, against a background of strong secular trends of increasing health promotion and declining risk factors, the overall program effects were modest in size and duration and generally within chance levels" (Luepker et al., 1994) The authors further concluded that "even such an intense program may not be able to generate enough additional exposure to risk reduction messages and activities in a large enough fraction of the population to accelerate the remarkably favorable secular trends in health promotion activities and in most coronary heart disease risk factors present in the study communities" (p. 1383).

Sanford Five City Project

The Stanford Five City Project took place between 1979 and 1992. The program involved the use of multiple media, educational, and health promotion activities to reduce risk factors including blood pressure, blood cholesterol, salt intake, smoking, physical activity, and adherence to antihypertensive medication regimens. A decrease in cardiovascular morbidity and mortality was observed during the intervention period; however, this occurred similarly in the control cities.

In summary, of the four public education efforts, the findings of the NHBPEP were most remarkable for achieving both a significant increase in awareness and a reduction in blood pressure. The program, however, currently functions at a lower level of activity than in the past. It was recently described as "a virtual program," with much of the educational materials and other resources provided online.[2] Results from the public education efforts in Pawtucket and Minnesota, although significant, were very modest and the Stanford Five City Project failed to detect significant differences between the intervention and control groups.

The VERB™ Campaign

The VERB™ campaign was an effort of the Centers for Disease Control and Prevention to increase and maintain physical activity among youth ages 9 to 13 ("tweens"). The campaign was conducted between 2002 and 2006 and involved the use of social marketing strategies such as paid advertisements, school and community promotions, and Internet activities. The campaign included television commercials as well as national print and radio advertisements. Advertisements were targeted to multiple ethnic groups, including African-American, Asian, Hispanic or Latino, and Native American audiences. The goals of the campaign were the following:

- Increase knowledge and improve attitudes and beliefs about tweens' regular participation in physical activity.
- Increase parental and influencer support and encouragement of tweens' participation in physical activity.
- Heighten awareness of options and opportunities for tween participation in physical activity.
- Facilitate opportunities for tweens to participate in regular physical activity.
- Increase and maintain the number of tweens who regularly participate in physical activity.

A 2005 study by Huhman et al. utilized a prospective, longitudinal, quasi-experimental design to determine the effects of the VERB™ campaign on physical activity among the target audience. Participants included 3,120 parent-child pairs. Baseline and follow-up surveys using random-digit dialing were used to measure the campaign's influence on awareness and physical activity. The authors found that after 1 year, 74 percent of children surveyed were aware of the VERB™ campaign—a 24 percent increase over the campaign's goal for the first year. Median free-time physical activity increased for several subgroups, including 9- to 10-year-old children, girls, children whose parents had less than a high school education, children in urban areas, and children engaging in low levels of physical activity at baseline. Among 9- to 10-year-olds, physical activity increased by 34 per-

---

[2] Personal comment by Dr. Ed Roccella in a presentation to the committee, June 2009.

cent compared to youth who were unaware of the program. The authors concluded that "promoting physical activity with child-focused commercial advertising shows promise" (Huhman et al., 2005, p. 277).

A recent report by the Institute of Medicine (IOM, 2009a) identified promising actions that local governments can take to prevent childhood obesity, and specified media and social marketing as a recommended action. Developing media campaigns and utilizing multiple channels to promote healthy eating and physical activity using consistent messages were recommended. The rationale supporting the goal and action step was based on the positive outcomes of the VERB™ campaign (Berkowitz et al., 2008), and research that shows that high-frequency television and radio advertising, as well as signage, may stimulate improvements in attitudes toward a healthy diet (Beaudoin et al., 2007).

RELATIVE COSTS OF POPULATION-BASED INTERVENTIONS

The comparative cost-effectiveness of population-based interventions compared to individual-level approaches to reduce blood pressure and cardiovascular disease risk has been the focus of researchers at the international level. Murray and colleagues conducted a review of the effectiveness and costs of a number of strategies to reduce blood pressure and cholesterol with the ultimate goal of reducing cardiovascular disease risk (Murray et al., 2003). They compared the effectiveness of four community-based interventions targeted at changing diets (salt reduction through voluntary agreements with industry, population-wide reduction in salt intake through legislation, health education through mass media, and a combination of salt intake legislation and mass media education) to individual-based interventions based on the pharmacological management of hypertension and cholesterol (individual-based hypertension treatment and education, individual treatment and education for high cholesterol concentration, individual treatment and health education for systolic blood pressure and cholesterol concentration, and absolute risk approach).[3]

The researchers found that population-wide interventions were more cost-effective than individual-based approaches. There was a 30 percent reduction in the salt content of food through legislative action and a 15 percent reduction in the salt content of food through voluntary agreements. The mass media campaign to reduce cholesterol through better diets and increased physical activity came in third. Based on the analysis, the

---

[3] The absolute risk approach consisted of providing individuals with an estimated combined risk of a cardiovascular event (35 percent, 25 percent, 15 percent, 5 percent) over the next decade above a given specific threshold of risk with a statin, diuretic, beta-blocker, and aspirin based on their risk level.

researchers suggest that population-based interventions could avert more than 21 million disability-adjusted life-years (DALYs). These interventions, although more cost-effective, have a smaller absolute effect on population health than individual-based strategies. Individual-based strategies, on the other hand, were shown to have a greater potential to reduce cardiovascular disease burden and improve population health, albeit at a higher cost. Pharmacological treatment based on the absolute-risk approach at a threshold of 35 percent risk would avert 65 million DALYs. This intervention was not as cost-effective as the population-based interventions. The authors suggest that a combination of population-based and individual-based strategies could lower the incidence of cardiovascular events by as much as 50 percent.

Palar and Sturm (2009) recently reported on the potential societal savings from policies that reduce sodium consumption in the United States. The researchers used the NHANES 1999-2004 data (blood pressure, antihypertension medication use, and salt intake) to model a number of sodium-reduction scenarios to determine the change in health care costs and quality of life that could be expected from a reduction in population-level sodium consumption. The scenarios simulated reductions in sodium intake from 3,400 mg per day to one of the following levels: 2,300 mg, 1,700 mg, 1,500 mg, and 1,200 mg per day. The model used dose-response estimates for sodium and hypertension reported in the literature to calculate changes in hypertension prevalence that would result from the associated decrease in salt intake (100 mmol reduction in sodium intake results in a 7.2 mm Hg reduction in systolic blood pressure and a 3.8 mm Hg reduction in diastolic blood pressure). The model input for annual hypertension costs per case was $1,598 (based on 2005 data) and is based on analyses of Medical Expenditure Panel Survey data for 2000-2003 (Trogdon et al., 2007).

The researchers found that lowering dietary sodium is likely to have sizable financial and health benefits. Reducing salt intake from 3,400 mg to 2,300 mg per day, for example, could reduce the number of individuals with hypertension by an estimated 11.1 million. A substantial reduction of salt intake down to 1,200 mg was estimated to reduce hypertension cases by 17.7 million. The annual, direct, health care costs saved related to a reduction in population sodium consumption was equally significant. The reduction from 3,400 mg to 2,300 mg of sodium per day was estimated to result in $17.8 billion (in 2005) in annual, direct, health care cost savings and a reduction of sodium to 1,200 mg per day was associated with an estimated $28.3 billion in annual, direct, health care cost savings. With respect to quality-of-life savings, the reduction to 2,300 mg of sodium per day was associated with 312,021 QALYs saved annually, and the 1,200 mg per day was associated with 496,897 QALYs saved. Finally, the value of the

QALYs saved with a reduction to 2,300 mg and 1,200 mg of sodium per day was $31.6 billion and $50.3 billion, respectively.

POPULATION-BASED INTERVENTIONS
AND HEALTH DISPARITIES

Not only are highly educated and affluent subgroups better positioned than the poor to benefit from innovations in medical care, they are also better positioned to respond quickly to public health messages and policies designed to either prevent or postpone lifestyle-related diseases such as hypertension. Hence, population-based interventions aimed at increasing physical activity and promoting healthy eating that fail to give due attention to differential response capabilities by race, ethnicity, socioeconomic position, and geographical location may inadvertently contribute to an increase in health disparities even as overall population health improves (Link and Phelan, 1995; Mechanic, 2007; Phelan and Link, 2005). Even if such increases in health disparities are time limited (i.e., returning to the baseline difference once disadvantaged populations make appropriate lifestyle adjustments), this nevertheless constitutes an unsatisfactory outcome if the objective is to reduce the overall population burden of hypertension while also reducing related health disparities.

Achieving these dual objectives will not be easy. A large and growing body of research (Acevedo-Garcia et al., 2008; Cutler et al., 1999, 2008; Massey and Denton, 1993; Williams and Collins, 2001b) documents that U.S. racial and ethnic minorities, especially African Americans and Hispanics, are overrepresented in urban areas that lack community-level resources to support healthy living. African Americans are simultaneously the most highly segregated racial group in the country (Acevedo-Garcia et al., 2008; Massey and Denton, 1993; Williams and Collins, 2001) and the group at highest risk for hypertension and its serious clinical sequelae. As discussed by Williams and Collins (2001), a high level of racial residential segregation can contribute to health disparities (hypertension and otherwise) through multiple pathways. These pathways include restricted opportunities for stable, meaningful employment that provides adequate family income and health care benefits; restricted access to high-quality, primary health care; restricted access to supermarkets containing fresh produce and foods low in sodium; restricted access to safe, well-maintained parks where residents can easily engage in regular, leisure-time physical activity; and finally, heightened exposure to air pollution, noise, and violence, which generate high levels of psychological stress.

More than 30 years ago, Harburg and colleagues (1973) were the first to demonstrate that mean blood pressures among African Americans in the city of Detroit varied with their place of residence. Specifically, blacks (especially black males under age 40) who lived in census tracts character-ized by high unemployment, low median household income and educational attainment, high rates of crime, and high rates of marital breakup had significantly higher age- and BMI-adjusted hypertension prevalence than blacks living in more socioeconomically stable census tracts (Harburg, 1973). Interestingly, the mean blood pressure of whites did not vary by residence in high vs. low "socio-ecological stress" areas, suggesting either a differential impact of socioenvironmental stressors on the blood pres-sure of blacks or substantive inequalities in the cut-points used to define "high"- and "low"-stress neighborhoods for blacks vs. whites in a place that was fast becoming the country's most racially segregated metropolitan area (Cutler et al., 1999).

The scientific literature documenting the relative lack of community-level resources to support healthy living in geographical areas characterized by low neighborhood wealth or high levels of racial residential segregation continues to grow. Morland and colleagues, for example, reported that the prevalence of supermarkets in the Atherosclerosis Risk in Communities Study increased linearly with increasing median home values and decreased linearly as the percentage of African-American residents increased (Morland et al., 2002). Franco and colleagues rated 226 food stores in Baltimore City and County on a healthy food availability index (HFAI) and found that HFAI scores were positively correlated with median household income of census tracts and inversely correlated with the percentage of African-American residents (Franco et al., 2008). Using data from the Multi-Ethnic Study of Atherosclerosis (MESA), Mujahid et al. (2008a) found that resi-dents in neighborhoods characterized by greater (self-reported) walkability, availability of healthy foods, aesthetic quality, safety, and social cohesion had lower BMIs (especially among women) than residents in neighborhoods with lower scores on these dimensions. Using this same indicator of neigh-borhood quality, Mujahid et al. (2008b) observed an inverse association between neighborhood quality and hypertension prevalence in the MESA sample; however, the association was significantly attenuated when race or ethnicity was controlled, suggesting that neighborhood social cohesion, safety, walkability, food availability, and so forth, may play an important role in racial or ethnic differences in risk of hypertension in urban settings (Mujahid et al., 2008a).

Compared to African Americans, disparities in hypertension and se-lected cardiovascular disease (CVD) risk factors by place of residence are less well studied in other racial or ethnic minorities. Again, using data from MESA, Osypuk et al. (2009) found that living in census tracts with higher proportions of foreign-born persons from China was associated with lower consumption of high-fat foods. Although living in census tracts with higher proportions of recent immigrants from Latin America was also associated with lower consumption of high-fat foods, residents of these census tracts reported significantly lower levels of physical activity. Osypuk and colleagues also found that residents of neighborhoods with higher proportions of foreign-born persons reported greater healthy food availability, but their neighborhoods were also reported to be less walkable, to have fewer exercise resources, and to have lower social cohesion. The researchers concluded that living in a contemporary immigrant enclave in the United States is not uniformly beneficial since these enclaves have varying patterns of healthy and unhealthy behaviors that can contribute to CVD risk (Osypuk et al., 2009).

Finally, in the Chicago Community Adult Health Study, Morenoff et al. (2007) found that mean blood pressure was inversely associated with neighborhood affluence (i.e., a concentration of well-educated residents with high-paying, managerial jobs). Although the prevalence of hypertension among blacks and whites was statistically significant even after controlling for individual-level income and education, adjusting for neighborhood affluence score completely eliminated this difference between the races. Interestingly, awareness of being hypertensive was greater in more disadvantaged neighborhoods and in areas containing large percentages of African Americans. Conversely, awareness levels were lower in neighborhoods containing large percentages of Hispanics and immigrants. After controlling for awareness, no differences in treated hypertension by race or ethnicity were observed; however, among persons taking antihypertensive medication, blacks were only 40-50 percent as likely as whites to be controlled. Neighborhood affluence did not modify hypertension control levels.

The above research findings of how mean blood pressures and hypertension prevalence vary within U.S. communities by race, ethnicity, and neighborhood affluence underscore the need to be attentive to the differential capacity of population subgroups to respond quickly and appropriately to population-based interventions aimed at reducing the overall burden of hypertension in this country. Healthy food has become increasingly scarce in many of our nation's older inner cities (Franco et al., 2008; IOM, 2009b; Morland et al., 2002; Zenk et al., 2005), where large numbers of new immigrants and historically disadvantaged native-born Americans (e.g., black Americans) live. Whereas the passage of national or state-level policies designed to reduce the exposure of Americans to foods high in sodium and increase their exposure to foods high in potassium will benefit all Americans to some extent, extra steps would seem to be necessary to ensure that residents in isolated, low-wealth communities benefit just as much as their wealthier counterparts. One example of a step in this direction is the CDC's partnership with the National Urban League's Health and Wellness Initiative (National Urban League, 2009) to increase access by African Americans and other inner-city populations to community-level resources (e.g., supermarkets, community gardens, safe places for physical activity, affordable primary health care) that would increase the capacity of these populations to fully benefit from a national hypertension reduction initiative. Similar opportunities are potentially available through other partnerships such as the Mexican American Grocers Association (BUSCA pique Network, 2004) to ensure that healthy, affordable foods remain available to the country's Hispanic population, especially in new settlement areas such as the U.S. South.

CONCLUSIONS

Based on the review of the literature there is strong evidence linking overweight and obesity, high salt intake, low potassium intake, unhealthy diet, and decreased physical activity to hypertension. These risk factors contribute substantially to the burden of hypertension in the United States; further, the prevalence of many of these risk factors is increasing. The observational and randomized clinical trial literature on interventions to reduce overweight and obesity, decrease salt intake, support eating a healthy diet, increase potassium intake, and increase physical activity also indicate that these risk factors are modifiable (Table 4.8) and that they can help reduce blood pressure levels. The committee concludes in light of: (1) the high prevalence of these risk factors that contribute significantly to the development of high blood pressure, (2) existing interventions to reduce these risk factors, and (3) the potential to reduce the burden of hypertension if the interventions are implemented, that actions to reduce these risk factors merit a high priority. Reducing heavy alcohol consumption was also considered; based on the low attributable fraction and the extremely low anticipated change in hypertension prevalence if heavy drinkers were to reduce their intake; it was not considered a priority for intervention to reduce hypertension.

DHDSP programs as described in Chapter 3 have focused primarily on secondary prevention activities and to a limited degree on the population-based approaches to hypertension. While secondary prevention is critical since it helps identify, treat, and rehabilitate people with established hypertension, stroke, and other cardiovascular disease, these activities should not preclude greater attention to conducting activities that prevent the onset of hypertension (primary prevention).

A stronger focus on primary prevention of hypertension is consistent with the DHDSP's responsibility as co-lead of Healthy People 2010 in achieving progress in reducing the proportion of adults with high blood pressure, and in increasing the proportion of persons ages 2 years and older who consume ≤2,400 mg of sodium daily. Broad primary prevention of hypertension is also consistent with the DHDSP's role as co-lead of the Public

Health Action Plan to Prevent Heart Disease and its recommendation for primary prevention activities related to children and youth:

Design, plan, implement, and evaluate a comprehensive intervention for children and youth in school, family, and community settings. This intervention must address dietary imbalances, physical inactivity, tobacco use, and other determinants in order to prevent development of risk factors and progression of atherosclerosis and high blood pressure.

The committee acknowledges that within the CDC, the DHDSP is not the focal point for addressing dietary imbalances, physical inactivity, and other determinants in order to prevent the development of risk factors and progression of high blood pressure. It also acknowledges that the focus of DHDSP activities is primarily adults, not children. The committee is aware that the DHDSP, through the Cardiovascular Health Collaboration of the National Center for Chronic Disease Prevention and Health Promotion, collaborates with units across the CDC. The committee believes, however, that this collaboration can be strengthened and extended to leverage the efforts and resources of those programs to ensure proper attention to the prevention of hypertension and the reduction of risk factors for hypertension.

4.1 The committee recommends that the Division for Heart Disease and Stroke Prevention integrate hypertension prevention and control in programmatic efforts to effect system, environmental, and policy changes through collaboration with other CDC units and their external partners, to ensure that population-based lifestyle or behavior change interventions where delivered, are delivered in a coordinated manner that includes a focus on the prevention of hypertension. High-priority programmatic activities on which to collaborate include interventions for:

- reducing overweight and obesity
- promoting the consumption of a healthy diet that includes a higher intake of fruits, vegetables, whole gains, and unsaturated fats and reduced amounts of overall calories, sugar, sugary beverages, refined starches, and saturated and trans fats (for example a diet that is consistent with the OmniHeart diet)
- increasing potassium-rich fruits and vegetables in the diet
- increasing physical activity.

4.2 The committee recommends that population-based interventions to improve physical activity and food environments (typically the focus of other CDC units) should include an evaluation of their feasibility

and effectiveness and their specific impact on hypertension prevalence and control.

The committee notes that, consistent with the DHDSP's focus on secondary prevention activities, its state program grantees have also focused heavily on secondary prevention.

4.3 To create a better balance between primary and secondary prevention of hypertension the committee recommends that the Division for Heart Disease and Stroke Prevention leverage its ability to shape state activities, through its grant making and cooperative agreements, to encourage state activities to shift toward population-based prevention of hypertension.

The committee finds the evidence base to support policies to reduce dietary sodium as a means to shift the population distribution of blood pressure levels in the population convincing. The newly reported analysis of the substantial health benefits (reduced number of individuals with hypertension) and the equally substantial health care cost savings and QALYs saved by reducing sodium intake to the recommended ≤2,300 mg per day, provide resounding support to place a high priority on policies to reduce sodium intake (Palar and Sturm, 2009).

The committee is aware of the congressional directive to the CDC to engage in activities to reduce sodium intake and the DHDSP's role in these activities. The DHDSP's sponsorship of an Institute of Medicine study to identify a range of interventions to reduce dietary sodium intake is an important first step. The committee believes that the DHDSP is well positioned at the CDC to take greater leadership in this area through it role as co-leader of Healthy People 2010, co-leader of the National Forum for Heart Disease and Stroke Prevention, and as the sponsor of grants to state health departments and other entities.

4.4 The committee recommends that the Division for Heart Disease and Stroke Prevention take active leadership in convening other partners in federal, state, and local government and industry to advocate for and implement strategies to reduce sodium in the American diet to meet dietary guidelines, which are currently less than 2,300 mg/day (equivalent to 100 mmol/day) for the general population and 1,500 mg/day (equivalent to 70 mmol/day) for blacks, middle-aged and older adults, and individuals with hypertension.

The committee recognizes other work in progress by the IOM Committee on Strategies to Reduce Sodium Intake; therefore, it did not develop recommendations for specific strategies to reduce sodium in the American diet.

4.5 The committee recommends that the Division for Heart Disease and Stroke Prevention specifically consider as a strategy advocating for the greater use of potassium/sodium chloride combinations as a means of simultaneously reducing sodium intake and increasing potassium intake.

As noted in Chapter 2, accurate information on sodium intake or the content of sodium in specific foods that contribute importantly to sodium intake is necessary for monitoring progress in its reduction. These data are not currently available in a systematic or timely fashion. The lack of data presents a significant gap that will hamper efforts to evaluate the progress made in reducing sodium intake in the American population.

4.6 The committee recommends that the Division for Heart Disease and Stroke Prevention and other CDC units explore methods to develop and implement data-gathering strategies that will allow for more accurate assessment and tracking of specific foods that are important contributors to dietary sodium intake by the American people.

4.7 The committee recommends that the Division for Heart Disease and Stroke Prevention and other CDC units explore methods to develop and implement data-gathering strategies that will allow for a more accurate assessment and the tracking of population-level dietary sodium and potassium intake including the monitoring of 24-hour urinary sodium and potassium excretion.

Possible concerns about the impact on survey participation in national surveys such as the NHANES could be addressed by sampling an additional small number of subjects who would be asked only for a 24-hour urine sample and basic demographic data.

The committee is concerned with the differential burden of hypertension among subgroups of the U.S. population as described in Chapter 2. It is equally concerned that some population-based interventions aimed at preventing or postponing the development of hypertension may increase health disparities even as overall population health improves. This is because some groups have a differential response capability to respond to population-based interventions related to their race, ethnicity, socioeconomic position, and geographical location. To assure that all Americans will benefit from population-based interventions, steps may have to be taken to target these populations specifically. Although the committee is not proposing a specific recommendation in this area, it strongly encourages the Division for Heart Disease and Stroke Prevention to build community partnerships that will help bring interventions to the populations who might need them the most, especially those in racial or ethnic and low-wealth communities.

The committee considered public education and social marketing campaigns as a potential priority strategy. The committee acknowledges the extraordinary progress that has been made to educate the public about hypertension. In the early days of the National High Blood Pressure Education Program, less than 25 percent of Americans were aware of the relationship between hypertension and stroke, and heart disease. Since that time extraordinary gains have been made in the population's awareness of hypertension; close to 75 percent of Americans are aware and 75 percent of Americans have their blood pressure measured every 6 months. Results to educate communities at the local level, however, have had mixed results; some changes in blood pressure were modest but statistically insignificant or did not endure over time. Sophisticated social marketing campaigns, such as the VERB™ campaign, are significantly more refined with social change theory underpinnings, targeting of audiences, and expectations for behavioral change than the earlier national and local education campaigns. Given the mixed outcomes associated with public education campaigns, the committee does not consider these efforts to be a priority for the DHDSP. Well-executed social marketing campaigns may have more promise; however, the committee believes that such campaigns should not be focused solely on hypertension. Rather, they should be integrated in general social marketing campaigns to promote healthy living through healthy eating and increased physical activity as suggested in the Institute of Medicine's 2009 report, *Local Government Actions to Prevention Childhood Obesity* (IOM, 2009a). The DHDSP's role, as suggested in Recommendation 4.1, would be to collaborate with other CDC units and external partners, to ensure that social marketing campaigns designed to promote healthy living also include a focus on the prevention of hypertension.

REFERENCES

Acevedo-Garcia, D., T. L. Osypuk, N. McArdle, and D. R. Williams. 2008. Toward a policy-relevant analysis of geographic and racial/ethnic disparities in child health. *Health Affairs* 27(2):321-333.

AHA (American Heart Association). 2009. *Make healthy food choices*. http://www.american heart.org/presenter.jhtml?identifier=537 (accessed November 5, 2009).

Anderssen, S., I. Holme, P. Urdal, and I. Hjermann. 1995. Diet and exercise intervention have favourable effects on blood pressure in mild hypertensives: The Oslo Diet and Exercise Study (ODES). *Blood Pressure* 4(6):343-349.

Appel, L. J., T. J. Moore, E. Obarzanek, W. M. Vollmer, L. P. Svetkey, F. M. Sacks, G. A. Bray, T. M. Vogt, J. A. Cutler, M. M. Windhauser, P. H. Lin, and N. Karanja. 1997. A clinical trial of the effects of dietary patterns on blood pressure. DASH Collaborative Research Group. *New England Journal of Medicine* 336(16):1117-1124.

Appel, L. J., F. M. Sacks, V. J. Carey, E. Obarzanek, J. F. Swain, E. R. Miller, 3rd, P. R. Conlin, T. P. Erlinger, B. A. Rosner, N. M. Laranjo, J. Charleston, P. McCarron, and L. M. Bishop. 2005. Effects of protein, monounsaturated fat, and carbohydrate intake on blood pressure and serum lipids: Results of the OmniHeart randomized trial. *Journal of the American Medical Association* 294(19):2455-2464.

Appel, L. J., M. W. Brands, S. R. Daniels, N. Karanja, P. J. Elmer, and F. M. Sacks. 2006. Dietary approaches to prevent and treat hypertension: A scientific statement from the American Heart Association. *Hypertension* 47(2):296-308.

Ard, J. D., C. J. Coffman, P. H. Lin, and L. P. Svetkey. 2004. One-year follow-up study of blood pressure and dietary patterns in dietary approaches to stop hypertension (DASH)-sodium participants. *American Journal of Hypertension* 17(12 Pt 1):1156-1162.

Armstrong, B., A. J. van Merwyk, and H. Coates. 1977. Blood pressure in Seventh-day Adventist vegetarians. *American Journal of Epidemiology* 105(5):444-449.

Ascherio, A., E. B. Rimm, E. L. Giovannucci, G. A. Colditz, B. Rosner, W. C. Willett, F. Sacks, and M. J. Stampfer. 1992. A prospective study of nutritional factors and hypertension among US men. *Circulation* 86(5):1475-1484.

Ascherio, A., C. Hennekens, W. C. Willett, F. Sacks, B. Rosner, J. Manson, J. Witteman, and M. J. Stampfer. 1996. Prospective study of nutritional factors, blood pressure, and hypertension among US women. *Hypertension* 27(5):1065-1072.

Beaudoin, C. E., C. Fernandez, J. L. Wall, and T. A. Farley. 2007. Promoting healthy eating and physical activity short-term effects of a mass media campaign. *American Journal of Preventive Medicine* 32(3):217-223.

Berkowitz, J. M., M. Huhman, and M. J. Nolin. 2008. Did augmenting the VERB campaign advertising in select communities have an effect on awareness, attitudes, and physical activity? *American Journal of Preventive Medicine* 34(6 Suppl):S257-S266.

Black, J. L., and J. Macinko. 2008. Neighborhoods and obesity. *Nutrition Reviews* 66(1):2-20.

BUSCA pique Network. 2004. *Mexican-American grocers association (MAGA).* http://www.buscapique.com/latinusa/buscafile/oeste/maga.htm (accessed November 5, 2009).

Cappuccio, F. P., and G. A. MacGregor. 1991. Does potassium supplementation lower blood pressure? A meta-analysis of published trials. *Journal of Hypertension* 9(5):465-473.

Carleton, R. A., T. M. Lasater, A. R. Assaf, H. A. Feldman, and S. McKinlay. 1995. The Pawtucket Heart Health Program: Community changes in cardiovascular risk factors and projected disease risk. *American Journal of Public Health* 85(6):777-785.

CDC (Centers for Disease Control and Prevention). 2003. *Early Release of Selected Estimates Based on Data from the January-March 2003 National Health Interview Survey.* http://www.cdc.gov/nchs/data/nhis/earlyrelease/earlyrelease200309.pdf (accessed April 13, 2010).

———. 2008a. *Alcohol and public health.* http://www.cdc.gov/alcohol/ (accessed November 5, 2009).

———. 2008b. *Prevalence of binge drinking and heavy drinking among adults in the United States, 1993-2007.* http://www.cdc.gov/print.do?url=http://www.cdc.gov/alcohol/data table.htm (accessed February 12, 2010).

Chien, K. L., H. C. Hsu, P. C. Chen, T. C. Su, W. T. Chang, M. F. Chen, and Y. T. Lee. 2008. Urinary sodium and potassium excretion and risk of hypertension in Chinese: Report from a community-based cohort study in Taiwan. *Journal of Hypertension* 26(9):1750-1756.

Cohn, J. N., P. R. Kowey, P. K. Whelton, and L. M. Prisant. 2000. New guidelines for potassium replacement in clinical practice: A contemporary review by the National Council on Potassium in Clinical Practice. *Archives of Internal Medicine* 160(16):2429-2436.

Coresh, J., D. Byrd-Holt, B. C. Astor, J. P. Briggs, P. W. Eggers, D. A. Lacher, and T. H. Hostetter. 2005. Chronic kidney disease awareness, prevalence, and trends among U.S. adults, 1999 to 2000. *Journal of the American Society of Nephrology* 16(1):180-188.

Croft, P. R., D. Brigg, S. Smith, C. B. Harrison, A. Branthwaite, and M. F. Collins. 1986. How useful is weight reduction in the management of hypertension? *Journal of the Royal College of General Practitioners* 36(291):445-448.

Cruz-Coke, R., R. Etcheverry, and R. Nagel. 1964. Influence of migration on blood-pressure of Easter Islanders. *Lancet* 1(7335):697-699.

Cutler, D. M., E. L. Glaeser, and J. L. Vigdor. 1999. The rise and decline of the American ghetto. *Journal of Political Economy* 107(3):455-506.

Dickinson, H. O., J. M. Mason, D. J. Nicolson, F. Campbell, F. R. Beyer, J. V. Cook, B. Williams, and G. A. Ford. 2006. Lifestyle interventions to reduce raised blood pressure: A systematic review of randomized controlled trials. *Journal of Hypertension* 24(2):215-233.

Dyer, A. R., P. Elliott, and M. Shipley. 1994. Urinary electrolyte excretion in 24 hours and blood pressure in the INTERSALT Study II. Estimates of electrolyte-blood pressure associations corrected for regression dilution bias. The Intersalt Cooperative Research Group. *American Journal of Epidemiology* 139(9):940-951.

Ebrahim, S. 1998. Detection, adherence and control of hypertension for the prevention of stroke: A systematic review. *Health Technology Assessment* 2(11):i-iv, 1-78.

Ebrahim, S., and G. D. Smith. 1998. Lowering blood pressure: A systematic review of sustained effects of non-pharmacological interventions. *Journal of Public Health Medicine* 20(4):441-448.

Elmer, P. J., E. Obarzanek, W. M. Vollmer, D. Simons-Morton, V. J. Stevens, D. R. Young, P. H. Lin, C. Champagne, D. W. Harsha, L. P. Svetkey, J. Ard, P. J. Brantley, M. A. Proschan, T. P. Erlinger, and L. J. Appel. 2006. Effects of comprehensive lifestyle modification on diet, weight, physical fitness, and blood pressure control: 18-month results of a randomized trial. *Annals of Internal Medicine* 144(7):485-495.

Forman, J. P. 2009. (unpublished). Data produced for the Institute of Medicine.

Forman, J. P., M. J. Stampfer, and G. C. Curhan. 2009. Diet and lifestyle risk factors associated with incident hypertension in women. *Journal of the American Medical Association* 302(4):401-411.

Franco, M., A. V. Diez Roux, T. A. Glass, B. Caballero, and F. L. Brancati. 2008. Neighborhood characteristics and availability of healthy foods in Baltimore. *American Journal of Preventive Medicine* 35(6):561-567.

Franco, M., A. V. Diez-Roux, J. A. Nettleton, M. Lazo, F. Brancati, B. Caballero, T. Glass, and L. V. Moore. 2009. Availability of healthy foods and dietary patterns: The Multi-Ethnic Study of Atherosclerosis. *American Journal of Clinical Nutrition* 89(3):897-904.

Friedman, G. D., J. V. Selby, C. P. Quesenberry, Jr., M. A. Armstrong, and A. L. Klatsky. 1988. Precursors of essential hypertension: Body weight, alcohol and salt use, and parental history of hypertension. *Preventive Medicine* 17(4):387-402.

Fuchs, F. D., L. E. Chambless, P. K. Whelton, F. J. Nieto, and G. Heiss. 2001. Alcohol consumption and the incidence of hypertension: The Atherosclerosis Risk in Communities Study. *Hypertension* 37(5):1242-1250.

Gelber, R. P., J. M. Gaziano, J. E. Manson, J. E. Buring, and H. D. Sesso. 2007. A prospective study of body mass index and the risk of developing hypertension in men. *American Journal of Hypertension* 20(4):370-377.

Geleijnse, J. M., F. J. Kok, and D. E. Grobbee. 2003. Blood pressure response to changes in sodium and potassium intake: A metaregression analysis of randomised trials. *Journal of Human Hypertension* 17(7):471-480.

Goldstein, M. 1990. The hypertension prevention trial. *Archives of Internal Medicine* 150(11): 2408-2409.

Graham, I., D. Atar, K. Borch-Johnsen, G. Boysen, G. Burell, R. Cifkova, J. Dallongeville, G. De Backer, S. Ebrahim, B. Gjelsvik, C. Herrmann-Lingen, A. Hoes, S. Humphries, M. Knapton, J. Perk, S. G. Priori, K. Pyorala, Z. Reiner, L. Ruilope, S. Sans-Menendez, W. S. Op Reimer, P. Weissberg, D. Wood, J. Yarnell, J. L. Zamorano, E. Walma, T. Fitzgerald, M. T. Cooney, A. Dudina, A. Vahanian, J. Camm, R. De Caterina, V. Dean, K. Dickstein, C. Funck-Brentano, G. Filippatos, I. Hellemans, S. D. Kristensen, K. McGregor, U. Sechtem, S. Silber, M. Tendera, P. Widimsky, A. Altiner, E. Bonora, P. N. Durrington, R. Fagard, S. Giampaoli, H. Hemingway, J. Hakansson, S. E. Kjeldsen, L. Larsen, G. Mancia, A. J. Manolis, K. Orth-Gomer, T. Pedersen, M. Rayner, L. Ryden, M. Sammut, N. Schneiderman, A. F. Stalenhoef, L. Tokgozoglu, O. Wiklund, and A. Zampelas. 2007. European guidelines on cardiovascular disease prevention in clinical practice: Full text. Fourth Joint Task Force of the European Society of Cardiology and other societies on cardiovascular disease prevention in clinical practice (constituted by representatives of nine societies and by invited experts). *European Journal of Cardiovascular & Rehabilitation* (14 Suppl 2):S1-S113.

Halton, T. L., W. C. Willett, S. Liu, J. E. Manson, C. M. Albert, K. Rexrode, and F. B. Hu. 2006. Low-carbohydrate-diet score and the risk of coronary heart disease in women. *New England Journal of Medicine* 355(19):1991-2002.

Halton, T. L., S. Liu, J. E. Manson, and F. B. Hu. 2008. Low-carbohydrate-diet score and risk of type 2 diabetes in women. *American Journal of Clinical Nutrition* 87(2):339-346.

Harburg, E., E. J. C., Chape C., Hauenstein L.S., Schull W.J., Schork M.A. 1973. Socioecological stressor areas and black-white blood pressure: Detroit. *Journal of Chronic Diseases* 26:595-611.

Hayashi, T., K. Tsumura, C. Suematsu, K. Okada, S. Fujii, and G. Endo. 1999. Walking to work and the risk for hypertension in men: The Osaka Health Survey. *Annals of Internal Medicine* 131(1):21-26.

He, F. J., and G. A. MacGregor. 2004. Effect of longer-term modest salt reduction on blood pressure. *Cochrane Database of Systematic Reviews* (3):CD004937.

He, J., M. J. Klag, P. K. Whelton, J. Y. Chen, J. P. Mo, M. C. Qian, P. S. Mo, and G. Q. He. 1991. Migration, blood pressure pattern, and hypertension: The Yi Migrant Study. *American Journal of Epidemiology* 134(10):1085-1101.

Heath, G. W., R. C. Brownson, and J. Kruger. 2006. The effectiveness of urban design and land use and transport policies and practices to increase physical activity: A systematic review. *Journal of Physical Activity and Health* 3(Suppl 1):S55-S76.

HHS (U.S. Department of Health and Human Services). 2008. *Progress review: Nutrition and overweight.* http://healthypeople.gov/data/2010prog/focus19/default.htm (accessed February 12, 2010).

HHS and USDA (U.S. Department of Agriculture). 2005. *Dietary guidelines for Americans.* 6th ed. Washington, DC: U.S. Government Printing Office.

Horvath, K., K. Jeitler, U. Siering, A. K. Stich, G. Skipka, T. W. Gratzer, and A. Siebenhofer. 2008. Long-term effects of weight-reducing interventions in hypertensive patients: Systematic review and meta-analysis. *Archives of Internal Medicine* 168(6):571-580.

Hu, G., N. C. Barengo, J. Tuomilehto, T. A. Lakka, A. Nissinen, and P. Jousilahti. 2004. Relationship of physical activity and body mass index to the risk of hypertension: A prospective study in Finland. *Hypertension* 43(1):25-30.

Huang, Z., W. C. Willett, J. E. Manson, B. Rosner, M. J. Stampfer, F. E. Speizer, and G. A. Colditz. 1998. Body weight, weight change, and risk for hypertension in women. *Annals of Internal Medicine* 128(2):81-88.

Huhman, M., L. D. Potter, F. L. Wong, S. W. Banspach, J. C. Duke, and C. D. Heitzler. 2005. Effects of a mass media campaign to increase physical activity among children: Year-1 results of the VERB campaign. *Pediatrics* 116(2):e277-e284.

IOM (Institute of Medicine). 2005. Dietary reference intakes for water, potassium, sodium, chloride, and sulfate. Washington, DC: The National Academies Press.

————. 2009a. *Local government actions to prevent childhood obesity*. Washington, DC: The National Academies Press.

————. 2009b. *The public health effects of food deserts: Workshop summary*. Washington, DC: The National Academies Press.

Ishikawa-Takata, K., T. Ohta, K. Moritaki, T. Gotou, and S. Inoue. 2002. Obesity, weight change and risks for hypertension, diabetes and hypercholesterolemia in Japanese men. *European Journal of Clinical Nutrition* 56(7):601-607.

Jalkanen, L. 1991. The effect of a weight reduction program on cardiovascular risk factors among overweight hypertensives in primary health care. *Scandinavian Journal of Social Medicine* 19(1):66-71.

John, J. H., S. Ziebland, P. Yudkin, L. S. Roe, and H. A. W. Neil. 2002. Effects of fruit and vegetable consumption on plasma antioxidant concentrations and blood pressure: A randomised controlled trial. *The Lancet* 359(9322):1969-1974.

Jones, D. W., and J. E. Hall. 2002. The National High Blood Pressure Education Program: Thirty years and counting. *Hypertension* 39(5):941-942.

Kaczynski, A. T., and K. A. Henderson. 2008. Parks and recreation settings and active living: A review of associations with physical activity function and intensity. *Journal of Physical Activity and Health* 5(4):619-632.

Kahn, E. B., L. T. Ramsey, R. C. Brownson, G. W. Heath, E. H. Howze, K. E. Powell, E. J. Stone, M. W. Rajab, and P. Corso. 2002. The effectiveness of interventions to increase physical activity. A systematic review. *American Journal of Preventive Medicine* 22(4 Suppl):73-107.

Karppanen, H., and E. Mervaala. 2006. Sodium intake and hypertension. *Progress in Cardiovascular Diseases* 49(2):59-75.

Kelley, G. A., and K. Sharpe Kelley. 2001. Aerobic exercise and resting blood pressure in older adults: A meta-analytic review of randomized controlled trials. *Journals of Gerontology. Series A, Biological Sciences and Medical Sciences* 56(5):M298-M303.

Klag, M. J., J. He, J. Coresh, P. K. Whelton, J. Y. Chen, J. P. Mo, M. C. Qian, P. S. Mo, and G. Q. He. 1995. The contribution of urinary cations to the blood pressure differences associated with migration. *American Journal of Epidemiology* 142(3):295-303.

Larson, N. I., M. T. Story, and M. C. Nelson. 2009. Neighborhood environments: Disparities in access to healthy foods in the U.S. *American Journal of Preventive Medicine* 36(1):74-81.

Lever, A. F., C. Beretta-Piccoli, J. J. Brown, D. L. Davies, R. Fraser, and J. I. Robertson. 1981. Sodium and potassium in essential hypertension. *British Medical Journal (Clinical Research Ed.)* 283(6289):463-468.

Link, B. G., and J. Phelan. 1995. Social conditions as fundamental causes of disease. *Journal of Health and Social Behavior* 80-94.

Lorenzo, C., M. Serrano-Rios, M. T. Martinez-Larrad, R. Gabriel, K. Williams, C. Gonzalez-Villalpando, M. P. Stern, H. P. Hazuda, and S. Haffner. 2002. Prevalence of hypertension in Hispanic and non-Hispanic white populations. *Hypertension* 39(2):203-208.

Luepker, R. V., D. M. Murray, D. R. Jacobs, Jr., M. B. Mittelmark, N. Bracht, R. Carlaw, R. Crow, P. Elmer, J. Finnegan, A. R. Folsom, R. Grimm, P. J. Hannan, R. Jeffrey, H. Lando, P. McGovern, R. Mullis, C. L. Peny, T. Pechacek, P. Pirie, M. Spralka, R. Weisbrod, and H. Blackblum. 1994. Community education for cardiovascular disease prevention: Risk factor changes in the Minnesota Heart Health Program. *American Journal of Public Health* 84(9):1383-1393.

Massey, D. S., and N. A. Denton. 1993. *American apartheid: Segregation and the making of the underclass*. Cambridge, MA: Harvard University Press.

Mechanic, D. 2007. Population health: Challenges for science and society. *Milbank Quarterly* 85(3):533-559.

Mensink, R. P., P. L. Zock, A. D. Kester, and M. B. Katan. 2003. Effects of dietary fatty acids and carbohydrates on the ratio of serum total to HDL cholesterol and on serum lipids and apolipoproteins: A meta-analysis of 60 controlled trials. *American Journal of Clinical Nutrition* 77(5):1146-1155.

Moore, L. V., and A. V. Diez Roux. 2006. Associations of neighborhood characteristics with the location and type of food stores. *American Journal of Public Health* 96(2):325-331.

Moore, L. V., A. V. Diez Roux, and S. Brines. 2008. Comparing perception-based and geographic information system (GIS)-based characterizations of the local food environment. *Journal of Urban Health* 85(2):206-216.

Morenoff, J. D., J. S. House, B. B. Hansen, D. R. Williams, G. A. Kaplan, and H. E. Hunte. 2007. Understanding social disparities in hypertension prevalence, awareness, treatment, and control: The role of neighborhood context. *Social Science and Medicine* 65(9):1853-1866.

Morland, K., S. Wing, A. Diez Roux, and C. Poole. 2002. Neighborhood characteristics associated with the location of food stores and food service places. *American Journal of Preventive Medicine* 22(1):23-29.

Mujahid, M. S., A. V. D. Roux, J. D. Morenoff, T. E. Raghunathan, R. S. Cooper, H. Y. Ni, and S. Shea. 2008a. Neighborhood characteristics and hypertension. *Epidemiology* 19(4):590-598.

Mujahid, M. S., A. V. D. Roux, M. W. Shen, D. Gowda, B. Sanchez, S. Shea, D. R. Jacobs, and S. A. Jackson. 2008b. Relation between neighborhood environments and obesity in the Multi-Ethnic Study of Atherosclerosis. *American Journal of Epidemiology* 167(11):1349-1357.

Murray, C. J., J. A. Lauer, R. C. Hutubessy, L. Niessen, N. Tomijima, A. Rodgers, C. M. Lawes, and D. B. Evans. 2003. Effectiveness and costs of interventions to lower systolic blood pressure and cholesterol: A global and regional analysis on reduction of cardiovascular-disease risk. *Lancet* 361(9359):717-725.

National Urban League. 2009. *Health and quality of life*. http://www.nul.org/what-we-do/our-programs/health-and-quality-life (accessed November 9, 2009).

NCHS (National Center for Health Statistics). 2003. *National Health Interview Survey (NHIS)*. http://www.cdc.gov/nchs/data/nhis/earlyrelease/earlyrelease200309.pdf (accessed February 12, 2010).

———. 2006. *Prevalence of overweight and obesity among adults: United States, 2003-2004*. http://www.cdc.gov/nchs/data/hestat/overweight/overwght_adult_03.htm (accessed February 12, 2010).

———. 2008. *Healthy People 2010 Progress Review: Focus Area 19: Nutrition and Overweight Presentation*. http://www.cdc.gov/nchs/about/otheract/hpdata2010/focus_areas/fa19_2_ppt/fa19_nutrition2_ppt.htm (accessed September 14, 2009).

Ohmori, S., Y. Kiyohara, I. Kato, M. Kubo, Y. Tanizaki, H. Iwamoto, K. Nakayama, I. Abe, and M. Fujishima. 2002. Alcohol intake and future incidence of hypertension in a general Japanese population: The Hisayama study. *Alcoholism, Clinical and Experimental Research* 26(7):1010-1016.

Osypuk, T. L., A. V. D. Roux, C. Hadley, and N. Kandula. 2009. Are immigrant enclaves healthy places to live? The multi-ethnic study of atherosclerosis. *Social Science and Medicine* 69(1):110-120.

Palar, K., and R. Sturm. 2009. Potential societal savings from reduced sodium consumption in the U.S. adult population. *American Journal of Health Promotion* 24(1):49-57.

Papas, M. A., A. J. Alberg, R. Ewing, K. J. Helzlsouer, T. L. Gary, and A. C. Klassen. 2007. The built environment and obesity. *Epidemiologic Reviews* 29:129-143.

Parker, E. D., K. H. Schmitz, D. R. Jacobs, Jr., D. R. Dengel, and P. J. Schreiner. 2007. Physical activity in young adults and incident hypertension over 15 years of follow-up: The CARDIA Study. *American Journal of Public Health* 97(4):703-709.

Pereira, M. A., A. R. Folsom, P. G. McGovern, M. Carpenter, D. K. Arnett, D. Liao, M. Szklo, and R. G. Hutchinson. 1999. Physical activity and incident hypertension in black and white adults: The Atherosclerosis Risk in Communities Study. *Preventive Medicine* 28(3):304-312.

Phelan, J. C., and B. G. Link. 2005. Controlling disease and creating disparities: A fundamental cause perspective. *Journals of Gerontology. Series B, Psychological Sciences and Social Sciences* 60 Spec No 2:27-33.

Poulter, N. R., K. T. Khaw, M. Mugambi, W. S. Peart, and P. S. Sever. 1985. Migration-induced changes in blood pressure: A controlled longitudinal study. *Clinical and Experimental Pharmacology and Physiology* 12(3):211-216.

Poulter, N. R., K. T. Khaw, B. E. Hopwood, M. Mugambi, W. S. Peart, G. Rose, and P. S. Sever. 1990. The Kenyan Luo Migration Study: Observations on the initiation of a rise in blood pressure. *British Medical Journal* 300(6730):967-972.

Rose, G. 1992. *The strategy of preventive medicine*: Oxford University Press.

Sacks, F. M., and E. H. Kass. 1988. Low blood pressure in vegetarians: Effects of specific foods and nutrients. *American Journal of Clinical Nutrition* 48(3 Suppl):795-800.

Sacks, F. M., B. Rosner, and E. H. Kass. 1974. Blood pressure in vegetarians. *American Journal of Epidemiology* 100(5):390-398.

Sacks, F. M., L. P. Svetkey, W. M. Vollmer, L. J. Appel, G. A. Bray, D. Harsha, E. Obarzanek, P. R. Conlin, E. R. Miller, 3rd, D. G. Simons-Morton, N. Karanja, and P. H. Lin. 2001. Effects on blood pressure of reduced dietary sodium and the dietary approaches to Stop Hypertension (DASH) diet. DASH-sodium Collaborative Research Group. *New England Journal of Medicine* 344(1):3-10.

Saelens, B. E., and S. L. Handy. 2008. Built environment correlates of walking: A review. *Medicine and Science in Sports and Exercise* 40(7 Suppl):S550-S566.

Schulze, M. B., K. Hoffmann, A. Kroke, and H. Boeing. 2003. Risk of hypertension among women in the EPIC-Potsdam Study: Comparison of relative risk estimates for exploratory and hypothesis-oriented dietary patterns. *American Journal of Epidemiology* 158(4):365-373.

Sesso, H. D., N. R. Cook, J. E. Buring, J. E. Manson, and J. M. Gaziano. 2008. Alcohol consumption and the risk of hypertension in women and men. *Hypertension* 51(4):1080-1087.

Sever, P. S., D. Gordon, W. S. Peart, and P. Beighton. 1980. Blood-pressure and its correlates in urban and tribal Africa. *Lancet* 2(8185):60-64.

Sondik, E. 2008. Focus area 19: Nutrition and overweight progress review. PowerPoint presentation at Progress Review Focus Area 19— Nutrition and Overweight, April 3, 2008, Washington, DC.

Stamler, J. 1997. The INTERSALT Study: Background, methods, findings, and implications. *American Journal of Clinical Nutrition* 65(2 Suppl):626S-642S.

Stamler, R., J. Stamler, F. C. Gosch, J. Civinelli, J. Fishman, P. McKeever, A. McDonald, and A. R. Dyer. 1989. Primary prevention of hypertension by nutritional-hygienic means. Final report of a randomized, controlled trial. *Journal of the American Medical Association* 262(13):1801-1807.

Stevens, V. J., E. Obarzanek, N. R. Cook, I. M. Lee, L. J. Appel, D. Smith West, N. C. Milas, M. Mattfeldt-Beman, L. Belden, C. Bragg, M. Millstone, J. Raczynski, A. Brewer, B. Singh, and J. Cohen. 2001. Long-term weight loss and changes in blood pressure: Results of the Trials of Hypertension Prevention, Phase II. *Annals of Internal Medicine* 134(1):1-11.

Stranges, S., T. Wu, J. M. Dorn, J. L. Freudenheim, P. Muti, E. Farinaro, M. Russell, T. H. Nochajski, and M. Trevisan. 2004. Relationship of alcohol drinking pattern to risk of hypertension: A population-based study. *Hypertension* 44(6):813-819.

Sturm, R., and A. Datar. 2005. Body mass index in elementary school children, metropolitan area food prices and food outlet density. *Public Health* 119(12):1059-1068.

———. 2008. Food prices and weight gain during elementary school: 5-year update. *Public Health* 122(11):1140-1143.

Thadhani, R., C. A. Camargo, Jr., M. J. Stampfer, G. C. Curhan, W. C. Willett, and E. B. Rimm. 2002. Prospective study of moderate alcohol consumption and risk of hypertension in young women. *Archives of Internal Medicine* 162(5):569-574.

The Trials of Hypertension Prevention Collaborative Research Group. 1992. The effects of nonpharmacologic interventions on blood pressure of persons with high normal levels: Results of the Trials of Hypertension Prevention, Phase I. *Journal of the American Medical Association* 267(9):1213-1220.

———. 1997. Effects of weight loss and sodium reduction intervention on blood pressure and hypertension incidence in overweight people with high-normal blood pressure. The Trials of Hypertension Prevention, Phase II. The Trials of Hypertension Prevention Collaborative Research Group. *Archives of Internal Medicine* 157(6):657-667.

Trogdon, J. G., E. A. Finkelstein, I. A. Nwaise, F. K. Tangka, and D. Orenstein. 2007. The economic burden of chronic cardiovascular disease for major insurers. *Health Promotion Practice* 8(3):234-242.

Wassertheil-Smoller, S., A. Oberman, M. D. Blaufox, D. Davis, and H. Langford. 1992. The Trial of Antihypertensive Interventions and Management (TAIM) Study. Final results with regard to blood pressure, cardiovascular risk, and quality of life. *American Journal of Hypertension* 5(1):37-44.

Whelton, P. K., J. He, J. A. Cutler, F. L. Brancati, L. J. Appel, D. Follmann, and M. J. Klag. 1997. Effects of oral potassium on blood pressure. Meta-analysis of randomized controlled clinical trials. *Journal of the American Medical Association* 277(20):1624-1632.

Whelton, S. P., A. Chin, X. Xin, and J. He. 2002. Effect of aerobic exercise on blood pressure: A meta-analysis of randomized, controlled trials. *Annals of Internal Medicine* 136(7):493-503.

Williams, D. R., and C. Collins. 2001. Racial residential segregation: A fundamental cause of racial disparities in health. *Public Health Reports* 116(5):404-416.

Witteman, J. C., W. C. Willett, M. J. Stampfer, G. A. Colditz, F. J. Kok, F. M. Sacks, F. E. Speizer, B. Rosner, and C. H. Hennekens. 1990. Relation of moderate alcohol consumption and risk of systemic hypertension in women. *American Journal of Cardiology* 65(9):633-637.

World Cancer Research Fund. 2007. *The choices that affect your cancer risk*. http://www.wcrf-uk.org/preventing_cancer/diet/choices_that_affect.php (accessed November 9, 2009).

Xin, X., J. He, M. G. Frontini, L. G. Ogden, O. I. Motsamai, and P. K. Whelton. 2001. Effects of alcohol reduction on blood pressure: A meta-analysis of randomized controlled trials. *Hypertension* 38(5):1112-1117.

Zenk, S. N., A. J. Schulz, B. A. Israel, S. A. James, S. M. Bao, and M. L. Wilson. 2005. Neighborhood racial composition, neighborhood poverty, and the spatial accessibility of supermarkets in metropolitan Detroit. *American Journal of Public Health* 95(4):660-667.

5

Interventions Directed at Individuals
with Hypertension

The previous chapter discusses population-based interventions that can be beneficial irrespective of hypertension status. This chapter focuses more narrowly on interventions directed at individuals who have been diagnosed with hypertension. A wide range of strategies are considered to reduce adverse health consequences associated with hypertension through early detection, treatment, and control. Strategies range from those that offer access to health care providers who screen and treat individuals with high blood pressure, reduce the cost of medications for those in treatment (insurance coverage, benefit design, cost sharing), support hypertension control (e.g., quality control measures), and increase hypertension awareness, treatment, and control (e.g., worksite wellness initiatives). The chapter also considers community health workers as a potential strategy to increase treatment adherence among individuals with hypertension.

ACCESS TO CARE AND CONTROL OF HYPERTENSION

Access to health care, including access to providers, is generally considered important to improved health outcomes (IOM, 2003b,d). Data are somewhat mixed, however, about whether hypertension control is improved if patients have a regular source of care (Ahluwalia et al., 1997; Col et al., 1990; Fihn and Wicher, 1988; He et al., 2002). Studies that have shown improvement in care include data from multiple surveys. For example, national survey data (e.g., the 1987 Medical Expenditure Panel Survey [MEPS]) have shown that having a regular source of care is associated with hypertension screening, follow-up care, and the use of medication (Moy et al., 1995). Data from the 1990 National Health Interview Survey (NHIS) showed a strong association between seeing a physician in the past year and taking action to control hypertension (taking medication, reducing salt, reducing weight) (CDC, 1994). Similarly, in an analysis of the NHANES (National Health and Nutrition Examination Survey) III, He et al. (2002) found that the percentage of persons with controlled hypertension was higher for those who visited the same facility (Odds Ratio [OR] = 2.77 [1.88-4.09]) or saw the same provider (OR = 2.29 [1.74-3.02]) for their health care. Another study reported that severe, uncontrolled hypertension was more common among Medicaid patients who could not identify a source of care (Lurie et al., 1984).

A few case control studies have reported similar findings. Shea et al. (1992b) found that severe, uncontrolled hypertension was more common among those who did not have a primary care physician (adjusted OR = 3.5 [1.6-7.7]) and those who did not comply with antihypertensive treatment (adjusted OR = 1.9 [1.4-2.5]). Ahluwalia and colleagues (1997) also found that controlled hypertension was associated with having a regular place of care (OR = 7.93 [3.86-16.29]. In a study of medically stable Department of Veterans Affairs (VA) patients terminated from regular outpatient care, compared with those retained in care, 41 percent of discharged patients had blood pressure that was uncontrolled compared to 5 percent at the time of discharge; blood pressures were taken 13 months after discharge (p < 0.001) (data for the control group were 17 percent at follow-up vs. 9 percent, a nonsignificant difference). Among discharged patients with diagnosed hypertension, systolic blood pressure rose an average of 11.2 mm Hg; diastolic blood pressure rose an average of 5.6 mm Hg (p < 0.001). Of the discharged group, 47 percent reduced their prescription medications compared with 25 percent in the control group (p = 0.002) (Fihn and Wicher, 1988).

Another study found that one of the factors associated with a hospitalization due to noncompliance with medication (medications included an ACE [angiotensin-converting enzyme] inhibitor) was the number of physicians seen regularly (p = 0.007). The adjusted OR for seeing a greater number of physicians was 2.0 (p < 0.005) (Col et al., 1990).

On the other hand, Kotchen and colleagues reported that neither having seen a provider within the past three months (p > 0.4) nor receiving care from the same provider at each encounter (p > 0.8) was associated with improved hypertension control (Kotchen et al., 1998). Similarly, Stockwell and colleagues found that a greater number of physician visits was not associated with awareness of hypertension, the number of antihypertensive drug days, or blood pressure control (Stockwell et al., 1994).

One of the reasons for the lack of a consistent association between access to health care and hypertension control may be because control of hypertension is inadequate even in those with access to health care. The NHANES III data have shown that 86 percent of individuals with uncontrolled hypertension have a usual source of care and average 4.3 physician visits per year; 75 percent of those who are unaware of their hypertension had had their blood pressure measured in the previous year. Lack of awareness of hypertension (OR = 7.69; p < 0.001) and being aware but uncontrolled (OR = 2.08; p < 0.001) were more likely in those ages 65 years or older, a population that has access to health care. In fact, most uncontrolled hypertension was mild systolic hypertension in older adults with access to health care and frequent physician contact (Hyman and Pavlik, 2001).

In a cohort study of a hypertensive VA population examined over a two-year period, less than 25 percent had adequate blood pressure control (<140/90 mm Hg), and 40 percent had blood pressure >160/90 mm Hg despite having an average of 6.4 (+3.3) hypertension-related physician visits. In addition, the mean systolic blood pressure (SBP) was virtually unchanged at the end of two years (146.2 and 145.4 mm Hg, not significant), while the diastolic blood pressure (DBP) decreased (from 84.3 to 82.6, p < 0.001) (Berlowitz et al., 1998). In the Stockwell et al. (1994) study of a well-insured population, 71 percent of individuals with hypertension were aware of their hypertension, only 49 percent were being treated, and only 12 percent of these were controlled (<140/90 mm Hg), despite frequent utilization of the health care system. Other researchers have also reported poor hypertensive control despite access to health care. Framingham study participants are highly compliant with follow-up exams, and findings on exam are discussed with them and also sent to their primary care providers. Still, in a Framingham cohort followed for four years, only 32 percent of untreated individuals with hypertension were subsequently on treatment, and only 40 percent of those not under control initially (>140 mm Hg SBP or >90 mm Hg DBP) were brought under control. Older age was a strong predictor for lack of control overall and among those under treatment (Lloyd-Jones et al., 2002).

In a survey of African Americans, 27 percent were unaware of their hypertension, despite 77 percent of them having had a blood pressure measurement by a physician within the previous 2 years; most had mild systolic hypertension. Those unaware of their hypertension were only slightly less likely to have had their blood pressure checked in the past year and were nearly equally likely as those who were aware to have had it checked in the prior 2 years (Pavlik et al., 1997). Kotchen et al. (1998) reported that only 70 percent of inner-city individuals with hypertension were aware of their hypertension, 55 percent were taking medication, and 26 percent were under control despite most having seen a physician within the previous 6 months.

Hyman and Pavlik calculated the attributable risk of lack of awareness of hypertension (Table 5-1): 46 percent of the attributable risk was being age 65 years or older; 22 percent was being male; 5 percent was being African American; and 9 percent was having no recent visit to a physician. They also calculated the attributable risk of being aware but having uncontrolled hypertension: 32 percent of the attributable risk was being age 65 years or older; 12 percent was being male; and only 8 percent was having had no recent physician visit (Hyman and Pavlik, 2001).

Consequences of Racial and Ethic Disparities in Awareness, Treatment, and Control

The above demographic differences in awareness, treatment, and control of hypertension directly contribute to the nation's long-standing racial, ethnic, gender, and age disparities from cardiovascular disease (CVD) and kidney disease. For example, using data from the NHANES III Mortality Follow-up Study (mean duration = 8.5 years; 143,551 person-years), Gu et al. (2008) observed a 3.86 greater risk (hazard ratio = 3.86, 95 percent confidence interval [95% CI]: 1.60-9.32) of CVD deaths among individuals with hypertension under age 65 compared to similar-age individuals with normal blood pressure levels. For non-Hispanic whites, the hazard ratio for hypertensives vs. normotensives was 1.70 (95% CI: 1.09-2.65); however, when non-Hispanic white hypertensives with controlled blood pressure were compared to their normotensive counterparts, the excess CVD mortality risk was no longer statistically significant (hazard ratio = 1.17, 95% CI: 0.72-1.91). For non-Hispanic blacks, a considerably smaller reduction in the hazard ratio was observed—4.65 (95% CI: 2.26-9.57) for controlled hypertensives vs. 3.93 for normotensives (95% CI: 1.78-8.68). The comparable hazard ratios for Mexican Americans were 2.09 (95% CI: 0.93-4.65) vs. 1.27 (95% CI: 0.46-3.52), a reduction slightly greater than that for non-Hispanic whites. Gu et al. (2008) speculated that the much smaller reduction in excess CVD mortality for blacks with controlled hypertension was probably due to several factors, including an earlier onset and greater severity of hypertension, less adequate blood pressure control, and less access to health care services. The cumulative effects of these factors probably led to more severe hypertensive target organ damage in blacks, thereby elevating CVD mortality rates even among those whose hypertension was controlled.

Lopes et al. (2003) described some of the most promising recent advances in nonpharmacologic (e.g., diet, physical activity) as well as pharmacologic approaches to treating hypertension in African Americans. First, they noted the acceptability (Vollmer et al., 1998) and the effectiveness (Svetkey et al., 1999) of the DASH (Dietary Approaches to Stop Hypertension) diet (low-fat dairy food, fruit or vegetables, and foods low in total and saturated fat) among African Americans who enrolled in the DASH clinical trial. Bray and colleagues, in an analysis of the effects of the DASH diet and three dietary sodium levels on blood pressure, also reported that the lower the sodium level, the greater the mean reduction in blood pressure. The effect was even more pronounced and beneficial for African Americans (Bray et al., 2004).

Lopes et al. (2003) also highlighted findings from a randomized controlled clinical trial (Kokkinos et al., 1995) wherein African-American men with stage three hypertension were assigned, or not, to a regimen of moderately intense, aerobic physical activity for 16 weeks. Engaging in aerobic exercise was associated with a significant decrease in blood pressure among the men randomized to the exercise arm. In addition, significant reductions in thickness of the interventricular septum and left ventricular mass, and in the left ventricular index, were observed for men assigned to the exercise arm. Collectively, these findings from well-designed and executed clinical trials of nonpharmacologic interventions for hypertension provide encouraging evidence that carefully supervised nonpharmacologic interventions focused on African Americans will likely reduce their excess risk for serious medical complications known to be caused by uncontrolled hypertension.

In summarizing advances in pharmacologic approaches to treating hypertension in African Americans, Lopes et al. (2003) concluded that studies continue to support the use of diuretics and beta-blockers as first-line antihypertensive therapy for everyone, regardless of race. However, they noted that findings from the African-American Study of Kidney Disease and Hypertension, or the AASK trial (Wright et al., 2002), also provided some support for the use of ACE inhibitors as first-line antihypertensive drugs in African Americans. An ACE inhibitor-based treatment program, they concluded, was more beneficial than calcium channel blockers and beta-blockers in reducing the progression of renal failure in blacks with hypertensive nephropathy.

Thus, recent studies indicate that closely supervised administration of nonpharmacologic as well as pharmacologic antihypertensive interventions by primary care providers could substantially reduce the black-white racial disparities in medical complications due to poorly controlled blood pressure. As is true of much of the extant literature on disparities in U.S. health care, the literature on hypertension continues to be disproportionately focused on blacks and whites and there is a lack of evidence-based recommendations that address disparities in hypertension awareness, treatment, and control for the nation's other high-risk populations.

TABLE 5-1 Proportion of Cases of Uncontrolled Hypertension in Each Population Subgroup Attributable to Identified Risk Factors

Risk Factor	Lack of Awareness of Condition			Acknowledged, Uncontrolled Hypertension		
	Relative Risk	Prevalence	Attributable Risk	Relative Risk	Prevalence	Attributable Risk
Age >65 (vs. <65)	7.69	0.13 + 0.0072	0.46	2.08	0.44 + 0.0153	0.32
Male (vs. female)	1.58	0.48 + 0.0046	0.22	1.30	0.43 + 0.0104	0.12
Non-Hispanic black (vs. non-Hispanic white)	1.45	0.11 + 0.0063	0.05	—	—	—
No physician visits in past 12 months (vs. >1 visit)	1.40	0.25 + 0.0062	0.09	1.89	0.10 + 0.0099	0.08

NOTE: Attributable risk is calculated as $P(RR - 1) \div [P(RR - 1) + 1]$, where P is the prevalence of the risk factor in the population and RR is the relative risk associated with the presence of the factor. Dashes indicated that non-Hispanic black race is not a significant risk factor in the model.
SOURCE: Hyman and Pavlik, 2001. Copyright © [2001] Massachusetts Medical Society. All rights reserved.

Physician Adherence to Guideline Recommendations and Hypertension Control

Although patient compliance with treatment is one reason for lack of hypertension control, it is also clear that lack of physician adherence to hypertensive guidelines is a major problem and a significant reason for the lack of awareness, lack of pharmacologic treatment, and lack of hypertension control in the United States (Chiong, 2008; Pavlik et al., 1997). Notably, older age and SBP predicted lack of control, even if the blood pressure was being treated (Lloyd-Jones et al., 2000; Pavlik et al., 1997). The NHANES III data show that lack of awareness of hypertension (OR = 7.69; p < 0.001) and being aware but uncontrolled (OR = 2.08; p < 0.001) were more likely in those ages 65 years or older: persons >65 years of age comprise 45 percent of the unaware, 32 percent of the aware but untreated, and 57 percent of the treated but uncontrolled hypertensives. Lack of hypertension control was associated with older age: OR = 2.43 (1.79-3.29) for ages 61-75 years, and OR = 4.34 (3.10-6.09) for those >75 years of age (Lloyd-Jones et al., 2000). In fact, most uncontrolled hypertension was mild systolic hypertension in older adults with access to health care and frequent physician contact. In addition, 75 percent of the unaware, 60 percent of the known but untreated, and 75 percent of the treated but not controlled hypertensives had a DBP <90 mm Hg (Hyman and Pavlik, 2001). A Framingham study found that only 33 percent were controlled to a systolic blood pressure goal, whereas 83 percent were controlled to a diastolic blood pressure goal. Of those on medication (61 percent), 49 percent were controlled to a systolic blood pressure goal compared with 90 percent to a diastolic blood pressure goal (Lloyd-Jones et al., 2000).

*Physician Nonadherence to Recommendations
for Treatment of Hypertension*

Systolic hypertension may be more complex to treat than diastolic pressure (SHEP Cooperative Research Group, 1991), but multiple studies show that physicians are unlikely to treat or intensify treatment for mild to moderate systolic hypertension (<165 mm Hg) if the DBP is <90 mm Hg (Figures 5-1 and 5-2) (Berlowitz et al., 1998; Hyman et al., 2000). Berlowitz and colleagues (in a VA cohort study) found that if SBP was >155 mm Hg and the DBP >90 mm Hg, treatment was intensified 25.6-35.0 percent of the time (the larger percentage was if the medication had been changed during the previous visit); if the SBP was >165 mm Hg and the DBP was <90 mm Hg, medication was increased 21.6 percent of the time, but if the SBP was <165 mm Hg, medication was increased only 3.2 percent of the time when the DBP was <90 mm Hg. Overall, treatment was

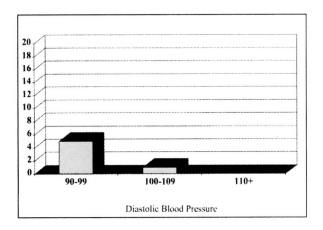

Diastolic Blood Pressure

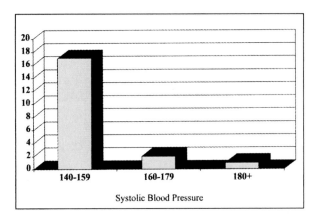

Systolic Blood Pressure

FIGURE 5-1 The proportion of patients over a 24-month period that was not diagnosed with hypertension, separated by average diastolic and systolic blood pressure.
SOURCE: Physician Role in Lack of Awareness and Control of Hypertension, Hyman, D.J., V.N. Pavlik, and C. Vallbona, 2000. Copyright © 2000 *Journal of Clinical Hypertension*. Reproduced with permission of Blackwell Publishing Ltd.

intensified in only 6.7 percent of visits (Berlowitz et al., 1998). Oliveria and colleagues also identified patients with uncontrolled hypertension. Pharmacologic therapy was initiated or changed at only 38 percent of the visits, despite documented hypertension for at least 6 months prior to the most recent visit (Oliveria et al., 2002).

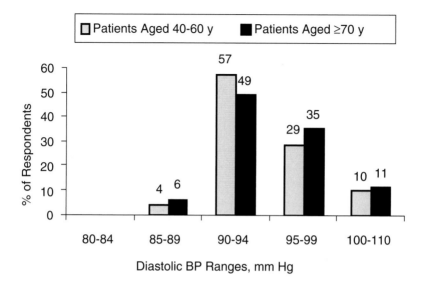

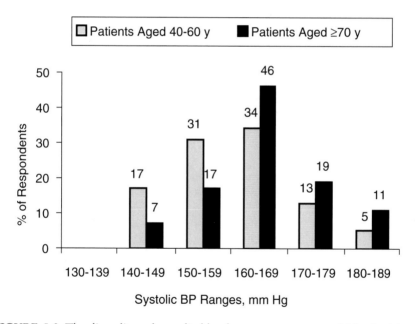

FIGURE 5-2 The diastolic and systolic blood pressure ranges at which physicians would start drug treatment in patients with uncomplicated hypertension.
SOURCE: Hyman and Pavlik, *Archives of Internal Medicine*, August 14, 2000, 160: 2283. Copyright © (2000) American Medical Association. All rights reserved.

In a study that linked adults' survey responses to their medical records, Hyman and colleagues found that these adults averaged 5.7 physician visits (median 4.0 visits). Of those with a 24-month average blood pressure >140/90, 25 percent were not diagnosed with hypertension. This proportion of "unaware" is comparable to the national rate reported by the NHANES III. Only 5 percent of those with a DBP greater than 90 mm Hg did not have a diagnosis of hypertension, but two-thirds were not diagnosed if the blood pressure was 140-159/<90 mm Hg. Of those on medication, the average blood pressure was 147/86, and only 24 percent had a blood pressure <140/90. When the DBP was >90 mm Hg, 98 percent had medication prescribed and treatment was intensified 24 percent of the time if the blood pressure remained >90 mm Hg. Treatment was intensified only 4 percent of the time when the SBP was >140 and the DBP <90 mm Hg. There was almost no action taken for persistently high SBP over many consecutive visits (Figure 5-1) (Hyman et al., 2000).

A recent study by Okonofua et al. (2006) assessed the extent of therapeutic inertia, defined as providers' failure to increase therapy when treatment goals are unmet, in 62 diverse clinical sites participating in the Hypertension Initiative medical record audit and feedback program conducted in the Southeastern part of the United States. The researchers found that antihypertensive therapy was not intensified in 86.9 percent of visits when blood pressure was ≥140/90. They estimated that improvement of 20 percent in the percentage of visits in which treatment is intensified, blood pressure control could increase from the study's observed 46.2 percent to a projected 65.9 percent in one year. The study did not provide information on the reasons for therapeutic inertia.

Physician adherence to guidelines for nonpharmacological strategies to manage hypertension is also problematic. Lifestyle modifications (weight management, healthy diet, exercise) or nonpharmacologic strategies have been found to be effective in managing hypertension as discussed in Chapter 4. Few physicians however, encourage patients to make such modifications. Based on data from the National Ambulatory Medical Care Survey (NAMCS) and the National Hospital Ambulatory Medical Care Survey (NHAMCS) for 1999-2000, only about 35 percent of patients with hypertension received counseling for diet and 26 percent for exercise (Mellen et al., 2004). Asians and Hispanics received the highest levels of counseling and non-Hispanic whites the least. Patients with Medicaid had the highest exercise counseling rates compared to patients with other payment providers. Diet counseling did not differ by payment provider. Diet counseling rates were also higher for patients with co-occurring diabetes, obesity, or dyslipidemia. With respect to exercise counseling, patients with obesity, had significantly higher odds of receiving exercise counseling. Patients with two or more cardiovascular morbidities were also more likely to receive diet and exercise counseling compared to those with less than one co-occurring morbidity. In NAMCS office-based practices, 36 percent of hypertension patients received diet counseling and 27 percent received exercise counseling. In NHAMCS hospital-based clinics, 25 percent received diet counseling and 14 percent counseling for exercise.

A more recent study found that health care providers fail to counsel patients with hypertension to increase physical activity as a measure to lower blood pressure. Halm and Amoako (2008), in an analysis of the NHANES III data, found that only one-third of patients with hypertension reported having received a physical activity recommendation from their health care provider. However, 70 percent of those counseled followed the recommendation and had on average a systolic blood pressure that was 3 to 4 mm Hg lower than those who did not follow the recommendation. Given the potential impact of nonpharmacologic strategies on hypertension management, this is an area that deserves greater attention.

Reasons for Poor Physician Adherence with Guidelines

Survey data shows that U.S. physicians are more likely to report that they adhere to diastolic threshold recommendations for initiating or intensifying treatment than for systolic thresholds (Chiong, 2008). In a national survey of primary care physicians, Hyman found that 33 percent would not start treatment for middle-aged patients with uncomplicated hypertension unless the DBP was >95 mm Hg; 52 percent of physicians would not start treatment for an SBP of 140-160, and 43 percent would not start treatment unless the SBP was greater than 160 mm Hg. For patients ages 40-60 years without complications who were on drug treatment, 25 percent of physicians would not intensify drug therapy for a persistent DBP of 94 mm Hg; 33 percent would not intensify drug treatment for an SBP of 158 mm Hg. Providers were even less aggressive in older patients: 48 percent would not take action for an elevated DBP of 94 mm Hg, and 67 percent would not take action for those ages 70 years or older with an SBP <160 mm Hg (Hyman and Pavlik, 2000).

Similarly, in a survey of primary care clinicians at three VA medical centers compared with the clinical database of patients cared for by these providers, clinicians overestimated the proportion of patients who were prescribed guideline-concordant medications (75 percent perceived vs. 67 percent actual, p < 0.001) and the proportion of patients who had blood pressures levels <140/90 at their last visit (68 percent perceived vs. 43 percent actual, p < 0.001). Physicians with lowest actual performance were the most likely to overestimate their adherence and rates of control (Steinman et al., 2004).

Oliveria and colleagues (2002) identified patients with uncontrolled hypertension. The treating primary care physicians were then asked to complete a survey about the patient visit (and given a copy of their office notes). The most frequently cited reason for no initiation or intensification of therapy was that there was a need to continue monitoring (35 percent); satisfaction with BP level (30 percent); it was not the focus of the visit (29 percent); the presence of a satisfactory DBP (16 percent); and the presence of only borderline hypertension (10 percent). For 93 percent of visits in which the physician reported being satisfied with the BP level, SBP was >140 mm Hg; 35 percent had a blood pressure >150 mm Hg; and the DBP was >90 mm Hg at 22 percent of these visits. Physicians attributed a higher risk to elevated DBP than to elevated SBP, and on average, physicians reported that 150 mm Hg was the lowest SBP at which they would recommend pharmacologic treatment for those without comorbidities (compared to 91 mm Hg for DBP) (Figure 5-3) (Oliveria et al., 2002).

In an older study in Wales, the reasons given for not starting or intensifying treatment in older patients with isolated systolic hypertension were fear that side effects would decrease the quality of life (39 percent); isolated systolic hypertension was an inevitable consequence of aging (35 percent); systolic hypertension was not as great a problem as diastolic hypertension (32 percent); isolated systolic hypertension was a compensatory mechanism to force blood through arteriosclerotic arteries (28 percent); and there was no beneficial effect of treating hypertension in the elderly (14 percent) (Ekpo et al., 1993).

Despite 1988 guidelines recommending treatment if SBP >140 mm Hg or DBP >90 mm Hg, 41 percent of primary care physicians had not heard of or were not familiar with the Joint National Committee (JNC) guidelines. Familiarity with the JNC guidelines was consistently associated with having more aggressive blood pressure goals, including statistically significant increases in initiating treatment for SBP in older patients and intensifying treatment for mildly elevated SBP and DPB in younger patients. However, familiarity with the guidelines was associated with a lower likelihood of intensifying treatment among older patients with mildly elevated SBP, particularly if they have isolated systolic hypertension (Hyman and Pavlik, 2000).

According to the NHANES III data, isolated systolic hypertension in the elderly comprises the majority of uncontrolled hypertension in the United States (Franklin et al., 2001; Hyman and Pavlik, 2001). Isolated systolic hypertension was also the majority subtype of uncontrolled hypertension among those >50 years of age. Additionally, only 29 percent of those with an SBP >140 mm Hg knew they were hypertensive, and 80 percent of both the untreated and the inadequately treated older individuals with hypertension had isolated systolic hypertension (Figure 5-4) (Franklin et al., 2001; Izzo et al., 2000). Factors that could lead to reduced control of

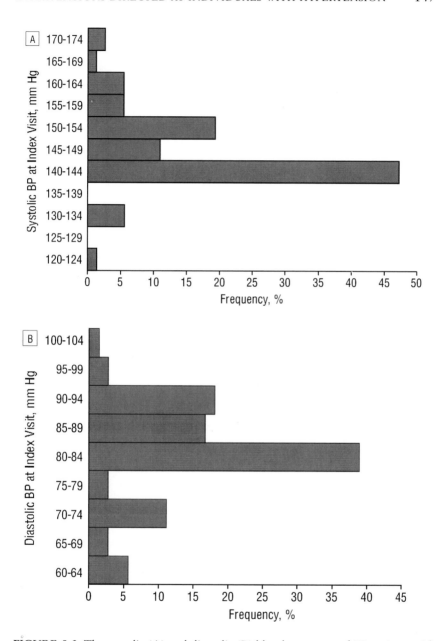

FIGURE 5-3 The systolic (A) and diastolic (B) blood pressures of 72 patients with no initiation or change in antihypertensive medication.
SOURCE: Oliveria et al., *Archives of Internal Medicine*, February 25, 2002, 162:417.

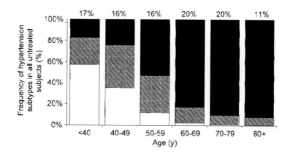

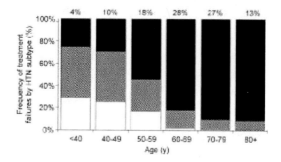

FIGURE 5-4 (Top) Frequency and distribution of untreated hypertensive individuals by age and hypertension subtype. Numbers at the tops of bars represent the overall percentage distribution of all subtypes of untreated hypertension in that age group. (Bottom) Frequency distribution of hypertensive individuals classified as inadequately treated by age and hypertension (HTN) subtype. Numbers at top of bars represent overall percentage distribution of all subtypes of inadequately treated hypertension in that age group. ■, Isolated Systolic Hypertension (SBP ≥ 140 mm Hg and DBP <90 mm Hg); ▦, Systolic-Diastolic Hypertension (SBP ≥ 140 mm Hg and DBP ≥90 mm Hg); □, Isolated Diastolic Hypertension (SBP <140 mm Hg and DBP ≥90 mm Hg).
SOURCE: Franklin et al., Predominance of Isolated Systolic Hypertension Among Middle-Aged and Elderly US Hypertensives. *Hypertension* 37(3):871.

hypertension in the elderly include potential biological resistance to therapy because of longer duration of hypertension and more target organ damage (Franklin et al., 2001; Izzo et al., 2000; Lloyd-Jones et al., 2002). However, it is also clear that physicians are less aggressive in treating older patients and less aggressive in treating isolated systolic hypertension (Berlowitz et al., 1998; Chiong, 2008; Hyman et al., 2000; Izzo et al., 2000; Lloyd-Jones et al., 2002). "Undiagnosed hypertension and treated but uncontrolled hypertension occurs largely under the watchful eye of the health care system"

(Hyman and Pavlik, 2001). Furthermore, physicians are not providing treatment consistent with the JNC guidelines, particularly in the treatment of isolated systolic hypertension, yet the largest attributable fraction for lack of awareness and lack of control of hypertension is being age 65 years or older and having isolated systolic hypertension.

Patient Nonadherence to Treatment of Hypertension

Patient noncompliance with prescribed antihypertensive medications is also a problem that contributes to suboptimal rates of blood pressure control. It is estimated that 50 percent of patients discontinue drug treatment after one year, and only 10 percent continue to follow advice concerning lifestyle modifications (Elliott, 2003). This problem can be addressed in part by increased attention from providers in identifying barriers to medication adherence and engaging patients in treatment decisions (Harmon et al., 2006). One study investigating how providers assess antihypertensive medication adherence revealed that patients were not asked about medication taking in 39 percent of encounters (Bokhour et al., 2006). Effective communication strategies and patient-centered counseling can be employed as a means to improve treatment adherence.

Krousel-Wood and colleagues (2005) suggest that future research should focus on the development of adherence models that consider the influence of social, psychological, and biological variables on antihypertensive medication adherence. Some established methods of improving adherence to long-term therapies include the provision of verbal and written instructions and patient education materials, simplification of regimen, once a day dosing (when possible), minimizing the number of pills, recommendation of well-tolerated therapies, and sensitivity concerning cost of pills and attempt to minimize out-of-pocket costs (Elliott, 2003).

Quality of Care and Performance Measurement for Hypertension Care

Shortfalls in the general quality of health care in the United States have been well documented (IOM, 2000, 2001b, 2003c). Studies discussed previously also indicate that the quality of care for hypertension received by some patients, particularly the elderly, is suboptimal (Oliveria et al., 2002). Further, the First National Report Card on Quality of Health Care in America published by the RAND Corporation in 2004 documented that patients with hypertension received less than 65 percent of recommended care (RAND, 2006).

Since the release of the Institute of Medicine (IOM) health care quality report series (IOM, 2000, 2001b, 2003c), improving quality of care has become of paramount concern for a whole host of health care system stakeholders (plans, providers, purchasers). In support of healthcare quality improvement, organizations such as the National Committee for Quality Assurance (NCQA) and the American Medical Association (AMA)-Physician Consortium for Performance Improvement (PCPI) have developed performance measure for determining benchmarks by which health care providers and organizations can assess their progress in improving health care services, processes, and outcomes. These organizations include specific performance measures for care of hypertension (Table 5-2). The Healthcare Effectiveness Data and Information Set (HEDIS®) performance measures put forth by the NCQA are widely used to assess quality of care and service of health plans. Health plans use HEDIS® results to determine the need for and focus of quality improvement efforts. In an analysis of the potential effects of eight HEDIS® performance measures related to the quality of care for cardiovascular disease and diabetes, Eddy et al. (2008) concluded that "[f]rom the perspective of the population as a whole, the most important single measure is the hypertension measure, which is very effective in reducing the risk of both MIs [myocardial infarctions] and strokes. This is due to the large number of people who had diagnosed but uncontrolled hypertension (approximately 14 percent of adults in the pre-HEDIS population) and the effectiveness of available treatments in preventing CVD events in people who have uncontrolled hypertension."

The PCPI is a physician-led initiative to develop tools by physicians for physicians. Members of the consortium include clinical experts representing more than 50 national medical specialty societies, state medical

TABLE 5-2 HEDIS® and Physician Consortium for Performance Improvement Hypertension Measures

Measures
HEDIS® Measures Controlling High Blood Pressure: Percentage of patients 18-85 years of age with a diagnosis of hypertension whose blood pressure was adequately controlled (less than 140/90 mm Hg) during the management year
PCPI Measures Blood Pressure Screening: Percentage of patient visits for patients aged 18 years and older with a diagnosis of hypertension with blood pressure recorded
Plan of Care: Percentage of patient visits for patients aged 18 years and older with a diagnosis of hypertension with either systolic blood pressure is greater than or equal to 140 mm Hg or diastolic blood pressure is greater than or equal to 90 mm Hg, with documented plan of care for hypertension

SOURCES: AMA, 2006; NCQA, 2009.

societies, methodological experts, the Agency for Healthcare Research and Quality (AHRQ), and the Centers for Medicare & Medicaid Services. The PCPI develops evidence-based clinical performance measures and outcomes reporting tools for physicians. Both organizations (NCQA and PCPI) envision that routine measurement of hypertensive care quality among provider groups or plans can lead to improved care processes and blood pressure control (Table 5-2).

Organizations or providers seeking to improve care processes, services, and outcomes can turn to a number of potential strategies. The AHRQ (2004) commissioned a review of the literature related to specific strategies for improving the quality of hypertension treatment. Among the quality strategies assessed were physician and patient reminder systems, continuing education for physicians, education for patients, and electronic transfer of patient data from specialty clinics to primary care physicians, among other strategies. The researchers found that most of the quality improvement strategies contributed to some improvement in the detection and control of high blood pressure, but it was difficult to determine which strategy was superior. The researchers also noted that multiple strategies are often used so it is difficult to identify which have the greatest effect on patient outcomes. The researchers observed that few of the quality improvement strategies had an impact on providers' adherence to optimal treatment guidelines. In summary, performance measurement can catalyze action toward quality improvement, some quality improvement strategies can improve hypertension detection and control, but improving physician adherence to treatment guidelines poses an elusive problem requiring further attention.

Cost of Medication and Hypertension

One reason for patient nonadherence with treatment is out-of-pocket costs for medication (Chockalingam et al., 1998). Controlling for health status, financial burden (out-of-pocket costs compared to income) has been shown to be significantly greater for persons with chronic conditions such as hypertension (Rogowski et al., 1997). Many studies, using a variety of methodologies, have documented a relationship between cost to patients, poorer adherence to treatment, and poorer control of hypertension (Fihn and Wicher, 1988).

Several studies have utilized survey data to assess the relationship between cost and adherence to treatment (Ahluwalia et al., 1997; Clark, 1991; Col et al., 1990). Generally these studies have reported that cost is a significant problem (Mojtabai and Olfson, 2003), particularly for ethnic minorities, those with lower incomes, and those with higher out-of-pocket costs (Fihn and Wicher, 1988; Steinman et al., 2001). In a 2002 nationally representative survey of chronically ill U.S. adults, 9 percent had cost-related antihypertensive medication underuse in the previous year, and 7 percent underused at least monthly. Income and high out-of-pocket costs (OR = 4.6; $p < 0.001$) were each associated with cost-related underuse of antihypertensive medications (Piette et al., 2004). In a 1981 survey, a larger proportion of people with uncontrolled or moderate to severe hypertension than controlled hypertension reported economic barriers to pharmacologic and medical care. Cost was a barrier to getting initial medication (36 percent for uncontrolled vs. 22 percent for those with controlled hypertension); medication refills (36 percent vs. 16 percent); and office visits (26 percent vs. 16 percent) (Shulman et al., 1986). In an older Gallup survey, 6 percent of respondents reported that they stopped their antihypertensive medication because they could not afford the cost (Gallup and Cotugno, 1986). A case control study found that control of hypertension was associated with reporting that cost was not a deterrent to buying medications (OR = 3.63 [1.59-8.28]) (Ahluwalia et al., 1997).

A few studies have looked at the cost of treatment and linked it to health outcomes. In the 2000 Health and Retirement Study, cost-related poor medication adherence was related to self-reported adverse health outcomes: 7 percent vs. 4 percent had worsening of hypertension (OR = 1.76; $p < 0.05$), and the odds of BP not being controlled were 1.92 ($p < 0.01$) (Mojtabai and Olfson, 2003). Noncompliance with antihypertensive medication is associated with increased hospital admissions (Maronde et al., 1989). McCombs et al. (1994) found that continuous antihypertensive therapy was associated with statistically significant reductions in hospital expenditures per patient that were greater than the accompanying drug costs; they estimated that an additional day of uninterrupted drug therapy would save $3 per day in total costs. In a study of medically stable VA patients discharged from regular care (compared with those retained in care), those discharged who reported a financial barrier to receiving care had a mean increase in SBP of 14.0 mm Hg and a mean increase in DBP of 6.4 mm Hg; this was significantly greater than the 3.2 mm Hg increase in SBP and 0.5 mm Hg increase in DBP among those reporting no financial barriers ($p = 0.001$ and 0.0001, respectively) (Fihn and Wicher, 1988).

Insurance Coverage and Control of Hypertension

One way of reducing patient costs of treatment is through insurance coverage. Many studies have examined the impact of insurance coverage on hypertension. Many of the data come from observational studies.

Insurance and Screening for Hypertension

Data from national surveys (1982 NHIS, 1987 MEPS) support the association of insurance coverage with hypertension screening, follow-up care, and use of medication (Chiong, 2008; Moy et al., 1995; Woolhandler and Himmelstein, 1988). For example, inadequate screening for hypertension was 18 percent among the uninsured vs. 11 percent for the insured (adjusted OR = 1.46 [1.28-1.67]; $p < 0.01$) (Woolhandler and Himmelstein, 1988). In another survey, the long-term uninsured (19.5 percent) and short-term uninsured (8.6 percent) were less likely than the insured (5.8 percent) to have been screened for hypertension in the previous 2 years (both were statistically significant differences) (Ayanian et al., 2000). In a randomized controlled trial that was representative of the U.S. population, the Rand Health Insurance Experiment, hypertensive individuals given free care were more likely to see a physician and to have their hypertension detected and a medication prescribed (Keeler et al., 1985, 1987).

Studies have assessed the impact of insurance coverage on utilization of antihypertensive medications (Adams et al., 2001b; Blustein, 2000). In a state survey among hypertensives, the adjusted odds ratio of prescription treatment for those with prescription drug coverage compared to those without prescription drug coverage was 1.20 (0.87-1.64) (Stuart and Grana, 1998). Data from the 2000 Health and Retirement Study showed that going from full coverage to partial coverage and from partial coverage to no coverage reduced compliance with antihypertensive medications (adjusted OR = 0.46; $p < 0.001$). The percentages with poor adherence due to cost were 11 percent for those with no coverage, 5 percent for those with partial coverage, and 4 percent for those with full coverage (Mojtabai and Olfson, 2003). Two studies used the 1995 Medicare Current Beneficiary Survey: Blustein (2000) reported that hypertensives without drug coverage (21.8 percent) were more likely than those with coverage (17.1 percent) to have not purchased any antihypertensive medication ($p < 0.01$); the adjusted percentage was 22.2 percent versus 16.9 percent (OR = 1.4; $p = 0.002$). Insurance coverage was not significantly associated with the number of tablets purchased in the unadjusted analysis, but in the multivariate analysis, medication coverage increased the number of tablets purchased per year by 37 ($p = 0.02$) (Blustein, 2000). Adams and colleagues reported that the utilization of antihypertensive medications was 1.26 ($p = 0.043$) among Medicare enrollees with coverage compared with those who had no coverage. Better insurance coverage led to greater use of antihypertensive medications and purchase of a greater number of tablets (Adams et al., 2001b). In a 2002 nationally representative survey of chronically ill U.S. adults, the OR was 3.3 ($p < 0.001$) for underuse of antihypertensive medication among those with no prescription coverage compared to those with such coverage (Piette et al., 2004).

On the other hand, in a study of low-income black and Hispanic patients diagnosed with hypertensive emergency or hypertensive urgency (compared to controls who were hypertensive patients hospitalized or seen in the emergency room [ER] for other acute conditions), Shea et al. (1992a) found that self-reported nonadherence to medication was not significantly associated with insurance coverage (OR = 1.6 [0.84-3.10]).

Some studies have assessed the relationship between insurance coverage and control of hypertension (Ahluwalia et al., 1997). An analysis of the NHANES III data showed that the percentage of persons with controlled hypertension was higher among those with private insurance as compared with uninsured or government-insured individuals (OR = 1.59 [1.02-2.49]) (He et al., 2002). In a survey of low-income African Americans, those having no insurance were significantly more likely to have uncontrolled hypertension (Pavlik et al., 1997). In a case series of consecutive hospital admissions, lack of insurance coverage for prescription drugs was associated with hospitalization due to medication noncompliance (medications implicated in hospitalizations due to noncompliance included an ACE inhibitor). The elderly (whose medications were not covered by insurance) were most likely to be noncompliant with their medication (52 percent vs. 31 percent; p = 0.04) (Col et al., 1990). Being switched from free care to paying $20-$30 per visit led to a significant worsening of hypertension at 6 months (10 mm Hg higher vs. no change in the control group) and one year (6 mm Hg higher than baseline [p < 0.001]). At 1 year, the percentage of people with a diastolic blood pressure <90 mm Hg was 51 percent, compared with 75 percent at baseline (p < 0.01); the percentage with DBP >100 mm Hg was 19 percent, compared with 3 percent at baseline (p < 0.01) (Lurie et al., 1986). Another study in two states assessed the relative risk of admission for avoidable hospital conditions (AHCs). The uninsured and those on Medicaid were more likely than the insured to be hospitalized with AHCs. For malignant hypertension, the odds of AHCs for the uninsured vs. those with private insurance were 2.38 (1.83-2.93; p < 0.05) in Massachusetts and 1.93 (1.41-2.44; p < 0.05) in Maryland. For Medicaid recipients, the odds ratios were 1.56 (1.29-1.82; p < 0.05) and 1.74 (1.36-2.13; p < 0.05), respectively (Weissman et al., 1992). A study of indigent inner-city hypertensive patients showed that hypertension control was associated with having insurance (OR = 2.15 [1.02-4.52]) (Ahluwalia et al., 1997). Another study of low-income black and Hispanic patients reported that severe, uncontrolled hypertension was more common among persons with no health insurance (adjusted OR = 2.2 [1.0-4.6]; p = 0.04) (Shea et al., 1992b).

The NHANES III data show that 92 percent of persons with uncontrolled hypertension have health insurance (Hyman and Pavlik, 2001). Similarly, among a well-insured population in New York, only 71 percent were aware of their hypertension, only 49 percent were treated, and only 12 percent had their blood pressure controlled at recommended levels (Stockwell et al., 1994).

Hypertension Control and Cost Sharing Among Those with Insurance

Cost sharing is described by AHRQ as the contribution consumers make toward the cost of their health care as defined in their health insurance policy. Rising health care costs have resulted in a shift toward greater cost sharing, particularly for prescription medications. There is a substantial body of literature (primarily observational studies) investigating the implications of cost sharing on medication utilization. Several studies have examined the impacts and health outcomes associated with cost sharing of "essential" medications such as antihypertensives.

A Cochrane review and other studies have reported that out-of-pocket costs (whether imposed as copayments, caps, ceilings, tiered drug categories, and/or restricted formularies) can reduce medication utilization, often substantially (Adams et al., 2001a; Artz et al., 2002; Austvoll-Dahlgren et al., 2008; Blustein, 2000; Cox et al., 2001; Fairman et al., 2003; Goldman et al., 2004, 2007; Harris et al., 1990; Huskamp et al., 2003; Kamal-Bahl and Briesacher, 2004; Landsman et al., 2005; Lexchin and Grootendorst, 2004; Motheral and Henderson, 1999a; Nair et al., 2003; Poirier and Le-Lorier, 1998; Reeder and Nelson, 1985; Schneeweiss et al., 2002a; Shrank et al., 2006; Solomon et al., 2009; Soumerai et al., 1991, 1994; Taira et al., 2006; Tamblyn et al., 2001; Tseng et al., 2004). In some cases, patients faced with out-of-pocket costs do not start their medication, reduce the amount of medication taken to make it last longer, switch medication, discontinue the medication, or take someone else's medicine (Cox et al., 2001; Schulz et al., 1995; Tseng et al., 2004). However, not all studies have shown significant impacts associated with cost sharing (Blais et al., 2001; Motheral and Fairman, 2001; Motheral and Henderson, 1999b). A review article, after excluding studies with very small cost-sharing changes and those without an adequate control group, estimated that cost-sharing increases of 10 percent would be associated with a 2-6 percent decrease in prescription drug use or expenditures (Goldman et al., 2007).

Most studies assessing the impact of cost sharing on essential drugs such as antihypertensives have reported a significant decrease in use (4-28 percent), with smaller impact seen for essential medications than nonessential medications (Adams et al., 2001a; Austvoll-Dahlgren et al., 2008; Goldman et al., 2007; Harris et al., 1990; Hsu et al., 2006; Landsman et al., 2005; Lexchin and Grootendorst, 2004; Motheral and Henderson, 1999a;

Nair et al., 2003; Reeder and Nelson, 1985; Schneeweiss et al., 2002a; Shrank et al., 2006; Soumerai et al., 1991, 1994; Tamblyn et al., 2001). A few studies, however, showed no significant difference in the use of essential drugs or between use of essential and nonessential drugs (Goldman et al., 2007; Johnson et al., 1997b; Lohr et al., 1986; Motheral and Fairman, 2001; Motheral and Henderson, 1999b). For example, Fairman and colleagues (2003) compared an intervention group of members switched from a two-tier to a three-tier plan with a comparison group retained in the two-tier plan (tiered plans employ formularies with differential copayments to encourage the use of generic drugs, or brand drugs that have been made available at a discounted rate). Although there was lower use of nonformulary (tier 3) medications in the first year, antihypertensive therapy continuation rates were not significantly different during the second year. Similarly, Motheral and Fairman (2001) found that moving from a two-tier to a three-tier plan resulted in no significant decrease in use of antihypertensive medication.

A Cochrane review concluded that the impact of cost sharing was greater for the chronically ill and persons on multiple drugs (Austvoll-Dahlgren et al., 2008). Most studies that have assessed the differential impact have found a greater impact of cost sharing among low-income patients (Brook et al., 1983; Goldman et al., 2007; Schneeweiss et al., 2002a; Shrank et al., 2006; Tamblyn et al., 2001), but not all (Poirier and LeLorier, 1998). It has also been reported that low-income patients were more likely than high-income patients to stop all antihypertensive therapy (Schneeweiss et al., 2002a).

Studies Assessing Impact of Cost Sharing on
Antihypertensive Medication Utilization

The impact of cost sharing specifically related to the use of antihypertensive medication has been assessed (Adams et al., 2001a; Blais et al., 2001; Blustein, 2000; Brook et al., 1983; Fairman et al., 2003; Goldman et al., 2004; Hsu et al., 2006; Huskamp et al., 2003; Johnson et al., 1997b; Kamal-Bahl and Briesacher, 2004; Keeler et al., 1985; Landsman et al., 2005; Motheral and Fairman, 2001; Motheral and Henderson, 1999a; Poirier and LeLorier, 1998; Schneeweiss et al., 2002a; Taira et al., 2006). In an analysis of the 1995 Medicare Current Beneficiary Survey, Blustein (2000) found that a $1 increase in out-of-pocket per-tablet cost resulted in the purchase of 114 fewer hypertension pills per year. In a study by Schneeweiss (2002a), 3 percent of individuals subject to cost sharing discontinued all antihypertensive medications; however, Johnson (1997b) found that the largest price increase led to fewer days of antihypertensive medication use, but not discontinuance of treatment.

In a cross-sectional study of Medstat's 1999 MarketScan database, Kamal-Bahl and Briesacher (2004) noted that the average annual use of antihypertensive medication was lower in the two- or three-tier plans with higher copayments, but not in single-tier plans. The average antihypertensive use in two-tier plans dropped from 18.9 prescriptions to 14.5 prescriptions with copayment increases of $5-$10 for brand-name products even though less costly generics were available. When brand-name copayments were increased to at least $14, the average annual use of antihypertensive medication fell to 10.8 prescriptions, despite a large increase in generic spending. The effect was greatest for angiotension II receptor blockers (ARBs) and ACE inhibitors.

Claims data have been used as a means to compare the impact of various benefit designs on the use of antihypertensive medication. Doubling copayments has been shown to reduce antihypertensive use by 26 percent, with less impact among those under regular care (Goldman et al., 2004). Higher cost sharing has been associated with delayed initiation of hypertensive therapy. Solomon and colleagues (2009) found that doubling copays led to initiation of therapy in 39.9 percent (compared with 54.8 percent) at one year and 66.2 percent (compared with 81.6 percent) by 5 years. The authors concluded that the effect of cost sharing is greatest soon after diagnosis and then declines over time; however, in those without prior medication experience it declines more slowly. Taira and colleagues (2006) found that medication compliance decreased substantially with increasing copayments.

In a study examining the effect of a preferred drug list restricting 17 antihypertensive medications, 21 percent of individuals on antihypertensives were found to discontinue their medication (Wilson et al., 2005). Another study found that a 66-100 percent increase in copayments led to a significant decrease in use of calcium channel blockers (CCBs) (4.1 percent) and ACE inhibitors (4.1 percent) and a nonsignificant decrease in ARBs (3.2 percent). There were also significantly higher discontinuance rates for ACE inhibitors (23.8 percent net increase) and ARBs (25.7 percent net increase) and a nonsignificant increase in discontinuance rate for CCBs in the three-tier plans (Landsman et al., 2005). In a prospective cohort study, Hsu et al. (2006) found that 15 percent of persons on long-term antihypertensive therapy whose drug benefits were capped were nonadherent the next year; significantly more than among those whose drug benefits were not capped.

Cost sharing is not always consistent with decrease in utilization. In one study, the intervention group with the change in benefits was less likely than the control group to stop using ACE inhibitors (Huskamp et al., 2003). In another study, the introduction of a new cost sharing led to a significant decrease in antihypertensive medication use at three months, but only a 1.1 percent decline (not significant) at 13 months (Blais et al., 2001). Fairman and colleagues (2003) compared those switched from a two- to a three-tier plan with those retained in the two-tier plan, and found that continuation rates for antihypertensive medications did not differ significantly at 6 through 38 months' follow-up. A RAND randomized controlled trial found that cost sharing had little impact on compliance with medication, but that those under free care were more likely to be taking medication (due to improved case finding, prescription of medication, and more frequent follow-up) (Keeler et al., 1985, 1987; Lohr et al., 1986).

Cost Sharing for Medication and Health Impacts

Although concerns have been raised about adverse health outcomes from reductions in "essential" drugs to treat chronic diseases, only a few studies have examined the impact of cost sharing on health outcomes, ER visits, or hospitalization (Adams et al., 2001a; Anis et al., 2005; Austvoll-Dahlgren et al., 2008; Brook et al., 1983; Goldman et al., 2007; Hsu et al., 2006; Lexchin and Grootendorst, 2004; Soumerai et al., 1991, 1994), and very few have specifically assessed the impact on hypertensive patients. Studies focusing on chronically ill patients have consistently shown greater use of inpatient and ER services with higher cost sharing; however, studies across broader ranges of drugs showed mixed results as to whether cost sharing leads to adverse health outcomes or increased costs (Goldman et al., 2007).

In a large study restricted to persons using medication for which a reduction in use might be expected to have an adverse affect on health, a 25 percent cost-sharing policy for prescription drugs up to an income-dependent deductible was associated with reductions in essential drug use and an increase in serious adverse events and emergency room visits among the elderly and welfare recipients. In contrast, reductions in use of less essential drugs were not associated with an increase in risk of adverse events or ER visits (Tamblyn et al., 2001). In a prospective cohort study, Hsu and colleagues (2006) reported that those whose prescriptions were capped had fewer office visits and worse physiologic outcomes (systolic blood pressure >140 mm Hg) than those whose prescriptions were not capped. Capped individuals also had an increase in ER visits, increase in nonelective hospitalizations, and higher death rates. The rates of elective hospitalization were not significantly different between the two groups.

In an older randomized controlled trial that was representative of the U.S. population (the RAND Health Insurance Experiment), those who had only catastrophic coverage had the highest blood pressures. Hypertensive individuals given free care were more likely than those under cost-sharing plans to be compliant with dietary recommendations, to have a BP <140/90 (43 percent in free care vs. 37 percent for those in a cost-sharing plan), and to have a BP <160/95 (65 percent vs. 56 percent). The impact was greater for those of lower socioeconomic status (SES). The authors estimated a 5-8 percent difference in the probability of death in the next year as a result of poorer hypertension control in the cost-sharing plan (Brook et al., 1983; Keeler et al., 1985, 1987). Hypertensive individuals in the cost-sharing plans were less likely to be diagnosed with hypertension despite having a blood pressure 4 mm Hg higher than those with free care who had also seen a physician This failure to diagnose and treat resulted in most of the overall difference in blood pressure control between plans at the end of the study (Keeler et al., 1985, 1987).

Not all research has demonstrated adverse health outcomes associated with cost sharing. For example, Johnson et al. (1997a) reported no consistent changes in office visits, emergency room visits, home health care visits, or hospitalization with copayment changes over four time periods. In comparing members switched from a two-tier to a three-tier plan with those retained in the two-tier plan, Fairman and colleagues (2003) found that the two groups did not differ significantly with respect to the number of office visits, emergency department visits, or inpatient hospitalizations. Another study assessing the impact of moving from a two-tier to a three-tier system also found no significant difference in emergency room visits or hospitalizations (Motheral and Fairman, 2001). A study comparing patients whose ACE inhibitors were put on reference pricing with those switched to an ACE inhibitor that was not subject to the price increase found a transient (2-month) increase in physician visits and hospitalization through the emergency room for those who were switched to reference pricing, but no evidence that reference pricing resulted in increased long-term health care utilization (Schneeweiss et al., 2002b). In a prospective cohort study, Hsu and colleagues (2006) reported that those whose prescriptions were capped had lower pharmacy and outpatient visit costs, but higher hospitalization costs and higher ER costs than individuals not subject to a cap. Total medical costs were comparable in the two groups. In a study of individuals who were switched to a no-cost ACE inhibitor compared with those who had cost sharing for ACE inhibitors, overall health care costs decreased (a slight increase in costs of physician visits but large decreases in medication costs) (Schneeweiss et al., 2002b).

EMPLOYER INITIATIVES TO ADDRESS HYPERTENSION

Traditional worksite health promotion programs strive to maintain worker health, improve work productivity, lower health care costs, and enhance organizational image and future interests (Goetzel and Ozminkowski, 2008). Increasingly, worksite health promotion programs are an element of corporate "health management" programs. Typically these programs provide a number of workforce-based initiatives that may include health promotion services, disease management, and other efforts to improve employee productivity by improving employee health (Goetzel et al., 2007).

Healthy People 2010 further describes workplace health promotion to include not only health education that focuses on skill development and lifestyle behavior change but also programs that help employees assess health risks and link to health plan benefits to provide appropriate medical follow-up and treatment. Key to these programs is their integration within the organizational structure and a supportive environment in which organizational values, norms, policies, and initiatives reinforce and support a healthy work culture (Partnership for Prevention, 2001).

The evidence supporting worksite prevention interventions is addressed in the Guide to Community Preventive Services (2009). The Task Force on Community Preventive Services reviewed the 31 studies to determine if health risks assessment with feedback plus health education with or without other interventions could lead to changes in employees' health outcomes; blood pressure was included among these outcomes. Of the studies reviewed, significant changes were seen in systolic and diastolic blood pressure. The median decrease in systolic blood pressure was 2.6 mm Hg, and the median decrease in diastolic blood pressure was 1.8 mm Hg. A decrease of 4.5 percentage points (median) in the proportion of employees with a high-risk blood pressure reading was also noted. The Task Force concluded that there is strong evidence of effectiveness to support worksite interventions that include the assessment of health risks with feedback plus health education with or without other interventions.

Worksite prevention programs may be attractive to employers if they can yield a return on investment (ROI). Koffman et al. (2005), for example, found a $3 to $6 ROI for every dollar invested over a 2- to 5-year period to implement a comprehensive worksite health promotion program focused on employee cardiovascular health. Aldana (2001) reported an average ROI of $3.48 in health care savings for every dollar expended on a health promotion program. Of the 12 studies reviewed to assess the financial impact of health promotion programs on health care costs, 7 studies had a positive ROI and 4 studies reported no effects of the programs on health care costs. Aldana (2001) also reported significant ROI (from $2.50 to $10.00 saved for every dollar invested) related to reductions in employee absenteeism.

Some employers have begun to explore benefit-based or value-based interventions as a means to address financial barriers that may hinder an employee's treatment. Benefit- or value-based insurance design refers to programs that provide a reduction in costs to targeted patients for targeted interventions that are deemed from the medical evidence to be highly beneficial. For example, a program might provide lower copayments for hypertension patients for blood pressure medications that are known to be effective (Chernew et al., 2007) Pitney Bowes, a Fortune 500 company, reduced or removed coinsurance on maintenance drugs for diabetes, hypertension, and asthma. Data available on diabetes care indicated that ER use decreased by 26 percent and pharmacy costs decreased by 7 percent. Total direct health care costs per plan participant with diabetes decreased by 6 percent. The hotel chain Marriott also began waiving employee copayments on generic drugs and reducing copayments by half for brand name drugs for diabetes, asthma, and heart disease (Capozza, 2008); health outcomes and other results are still pending.

To promote worksite wellness, the Centers for Disease Control and Prevention (CDC) Division for Heart Disease and Stroke Prevention (DHDSP) has partnered with the National Business Coalition on Health, the National Business Group on Health (NBGH), and other private entities. In 2006, NBGH released *A Purchaser's Guide to Clinical Preventive Services: Moving Science into Coverage* developed in cooperation with the CDC and the AHRQ (CDC and NBGH, 2006). The guide provides advice to employers to assist them in purchasing health services that have the greatest impact on health improvement and are cost-effective. Hypertension screening, counseling, and treatment are identified among the top 25 high-value preventive services identified in the guide. The document ranked hypertension screening, counseling, and treatment with the highest score of clinical preventive burden of disease (on a scale of 1 to 5 where 5 is the highest score) and a medium score of 3 for cost-effectiveness (on the 5-point scale). Overall, hypertension screening, counseling, and treatment was ranked sixth out of the top 25 high-value preventive services (CDC, 2009; Maciosek et al., 2006; Partnership for Prevention, 2006).

Other products useful for employers include the CDC's Successful Business Strategies to Prevent Heart Disease and Stroke Toolkit, which provides guidance and resources to be used by state heart disease and stroke prevention programs to engage the business community (CDC, 2008b). The toolkit includes a check list to help employers choose and negotiate health benefit packages that fit the needs of their employees. The American College of Sport Medicine's Worksite Health Handbook is another resource for employers. It provides a compilation of research, evidence, and practice information that supports worksite health promotion as a means to enhance productivity management, health promotion, and chronic disease management (American College of Sports Medicine, 2009).

COMMUNITY HEALTH WORKERS AND HYPERTENSION

Previous sections have addressed a number of system factors that influence the control of hypertension. Individual factors such as motivation to take prescribed medication and healthy lifestyle choices also play a role. Community health workers (CHWs) have been studied as a strategy to help improve hypertension control (Brownstein et al., 2005, 2007). Community health workers are broadly defined as "community members who work almost exclusively in community settings and who serve as connectors between healthcare consumers and providers to promote health among groups that have traditionally lacked access to care" (Witmer et al., 1995). They serve as lay educators, coaches, navigators, advocates, and liaisons to the health care system (Brownstein et al., 2005).

Brownstein et al. (2007) reviewed randomized controlled trials (RCTs) and other studies to examine the effectiveness of CHWs in supporting the care of individuals with hypertension. Highlights from the review include positive behavioral changes in 9 of 10 studies: improved appointment keeping, improved adherence to medications, and improved blood pressure control. Among the 5 studies that addressed adherence to medications, 2 RCTs saw significant improvement in the intervention groups that included CHWs compared to the control group. Another RCT found 26 percent greater compliance among patients receiving intense CHW interventions. A time-series study and a before-and-after study also noted improvement with CHW interventions. With respect to blood pressure control, 9 of 10 studies reported positive improvements. Improvement in blood pressure control ranged from 4 to 46 percent over different time periods (6 to 24 months). One study did not find differences between CHW and control groups.

The roles and duties of CHWs tend to be similar across studies and reflect the common objective of improving blood pressure control through a range of physician- or nurse-supervised behavioral and social support interventions. The latter typically include measuring and monitoring blood pressure; providing health education to patients and families about behavioral risk factors for hypertension; recommending changes in diet and physical activity; explaining treatment protocols, health insurance matters, and the importance of adhering to medication regimens; providing help with obtaining transportation to medical appointments; serving as mediators between patients and health care and social service systems; arranging for translation services; and finally, listening to patients and their family members, motivating them, reducing their isolation, and leading self-help groups.

Some of the roles and the successes achieved appear to be similar to those of nurses who have provided educational interventions aimed at hypertension control and suggest an efficient strategy for bringing about enhanced treatment and sustained blood pressure control for targeted racially or ethnically diverse, high-risk populations. Although trained laypeople cannot perform in the same capacity as professional nurses and health educators, with appropriate training and supervision they can successfully contribute to the care of community members with hypertension (Bosworth et al., 2005).

Community health workers may also play an important role in linking diverse communities to the health care system (HRSA, 2007; IOM, 2003e). The IOM committee that produced the report *Unequal Treatment: Confronting Racial and Ethnic Disparities in Health Care* found that "community health workers offer promise as a community-based resource to increase racial and ethnic minorities' access to healthcare and to serve as a liaison between healthcare providers and the communities they serve." Based on this finding, the committee recommended supporting the use of community health workers. "Programs to support the use of community health workers (e.g., as healthcare navigators), especially among medically underserved and racial and ethnic minority populations, should be expanded, evaluated, and replicated" (IOM, 2003e, p. 195).

Federal agencies, including the CDC and the National Heart, Lung, and Blood Institute, recognize the potential contributions of CHWs in the prevention and control of cardiovascular disease, including hypertension. Training manuals for community health workers and lay health educators have been developed and disseminated by these agencies (CDC, 2008a; NHLBI, 2006a,b, 2007, 2008a,b).

CONCLUSIONS

Access to health care and the quality of health care have been areas of serious review and analysis at the Institute of Medicine. In the early 2000s, the IOM produced a series of reports on the general benefits of having health insurance and the adverse health consequences when insurance is lacking (IOM, 2001a, 2002a,b, 2003b,d, 2004). The IOM also published landmark reports on the poor state of quality in the health care delivery system and on a comprehensive vision for how the health care system might be transformed to be safe, effective, patient-centered, timely, efficient, and equitable (IOM, 2001b, 2003c). These reports do not specifically address access to hypertension care or providers. One report, *Priority Areas for National Action: Transforming Health Care Quality* (IOM, 2003c), however, identified hypertension (with a focus on appropriate management of early disease) as one of 20 priority areas for improvement in health care quality.

The committee, in its review of the evidence related to hypertension control and access to care and providers, found that although lack of health insurance is associated with poorer screening rates, poorer compliance with medication, and poorer blood pressure control; the vast majority of individuals with uncontrolled hypertension in the United States are insured. In fact, the committee found that lack of health insurance or lack of access to health care accounts for a relatively low proportion of poor awareness or poor control of hypertension. Within the context of the current health care reform debate, the committee supports the recommendations by a former IOM committee for "comprehensive and affordable health care to every person residing in the United States" and that "all public and privately funded insurance include appropriate preventive services as recommended by the U.S. Preventive Services Task Force" (IOM, 2003a). The committee encourages the Division for Heart Disease and Stroke Prevention to be supportive of such efforts but directs the division's attention to addressing the quality of care for hypertension, especially as it relates to health care providers' capacity to deliver quality hypertensive care.

Based on the review of the literature, there is strong evidence that physicians are not paying adequate attention to treating and controlling systolic hypertension. The goal of improving the education and training of health care providers in the prevention of cardiovascular disease is central to the Public Health Action Plan to Prevent Heart Disease and Stroke, the DHDSP Strategic Plan, and the National Heart Disease and Stroke Prevention Program (as described in Chapter 3). For example, under the National Heart Disease and Stroke Prevention Program, Virginia, Georgia, and South Carolina have programs to support professional education and training to promote quality health care.[1] The committee believes that understanding the reasons behind nonadherence and increasing physician awareness, understanding, and implementation of JNC treatment guidelines are essential to increasing the number of individuals with controlled hypertension, especially systolic hypertension. This is especially salient among the elderly, given the aging of the U.S. population. The committee is concerned that undiagnosed hypertension and treated but uncontrolled hypertension are occurring under "the watchful eye of the health care system" and that physicians are not adhering to JNC guidelines. While a number of studies have documented the problem, little information is available to understand clearly why providers do not adhere to JNC guidelines related to screening and treating or intensifying treatment for mild to moderate systolic hypertension. As one study reported, some physicians were satisfied with blood pressure levels above 140 mm Hg and 90 mm Hg, and some physicians attributed higher risk to elevated diastolic pressure than to elevated systolic pressure, especially in the elderly (Oliveria et al., 2002). Numerous ques-

---

[1] Virginia's program primarily focuses on educating, training, and certifying health care professionals in the proper procedures in measuring blood pressure. The Georgia Cardiovascular Health Initiative, along with its partner, the International Society on Hypertension in Blacks, conducts a series of continuing medical education for community-based health center staff and other providers. Similarly, South Carolina and its partner, the American Society of Hypertension, Inc., provide continuing medical education to health professionals on evidence-based treatment of hypertension. The training leads to certification as a "hypertension expert."

tions remain regarding whether the lack of adherence is related to a lack of physician agreement with the new treatment guidelines, physician lack of knowledge regarding the guidelines, inertia due to treating at the previous guideline of 160/95 mm Hg, or other barriers.

5.1 The committee recommends that the Division for Heart Disease and Stroke Prevention give high priority to conducting research to better understand the reasons behind poor physician adherence to current JNC guidelines. Once these factors are better understood, strategies should be developed to increase the likelihood that primary providers will screen for and treat hypertension appropriately, especially in elderly patients.

Educating clinicians about the importance of treating and controlling systolic hypertension may be one important strategy but is not expected to be the only one.

Furthermore, high levels of uncontrolled hypertension are indicative of poor-quality care. The committee agrees with the IOM recommendation that identified hypertension (with a special focus on appropriate management of early disease) as one of the top 20 priorities for improvement in health care quality (IOM, 2003c). The evidence reviewed indicates that although physicians screen for blood pressure, screening does not always lead to treatment or to intensified treatment when appropriate.

5.2 The committee recommends that the Division for Heart Disease and Stroke Prevention work with the Joint Commission and the health care quality community to improve provider performance on measures focused on assessing adherence to guidelines for screening for hypertension, the development of a hypertension disease management plan that is consistent with JNC guidelines, and achievement of blood pressure control.

Out-of-pocket cost of medication has been identified in the literature as a significant barrier to patient adherence with hypertension treatment. It is estimated that for every 10 percent increase in cost sharing, overall prescription drug spending decreases by 2-6 percent (Goldman et al., 2007). Goldman and colleagues compared the impact of reducing cost barriers with other interventions designed to improve adherence with medications for chronic conditions and noted that even the most successful interventions designed to increase patient adherence to medication did not result in larger improvements in adherence than reducing the costs, and generally relied on complicated, labor-intensive regimens (Goldman et al., 2007).

The committee finds the evidence convincing that reducing costs of antihypertensive medication is an important and efficient way to increase medication adherence.

5.3 The committee recommends that the Division for Heart Disease and Stroke Prevention should encourage the Centers for Medicare & Medicaid Services to recommend the elimination or reduction of deductibles for antihypertensive medications among plans participating under Medicare Part D, and work with state Medicaid programs and encourage them to eliminate deductibles and copayment for antihypertensive medications. The committee also recommends that the DHDSP work with the pharmaceutical industry and its trade organizations to standardize and simplify applications for patient assistance programs that provide reduced-cost or free antihypertensive medications for low-income, underinsured, or uninsured individuals.

The committee notes that the DHDSP is also well positioned to educate the private sector that eliminating or reducing the costs of antihypertensive medications is an important and efficient way to increase medication adherence. Through collaborations with the National Forum for Heart Disease and Stroke Prevention (Chapter 3) and cooperative agreements and partnerships with the private sector, the division provides support and guidance to the employer community on hypertension and cardiovascular disease prevention and control. The division's product, The Business of Heart Disease and Stroke Prevention Toolkit, for example, although extremely informative and useful, does not address benefit or value-based benefit purchasing that can help reduce costs of essential antihypertensive medications. The private sector is already experimenting with reducing the copayments associated with drugs commonly prescribed for diabetes, asthma, and hypertension (Pitney Bowes, Marriott, others). The results of these experiments should be shared broadly with the business community.

5.4 The committee recommends that the Division for Heart Disease and Stroke Prevention collaborate with leaders in the business community to educate them about the impact of reduced patient costs on antihypertensive medication adherence and work with them to encourage employers to leverage their health care purchasing power to advocate for reduced deductibles and copayments for antihypertensive medications in their health insurance benefits packages.

The DHDSP might also consider working with the business community to evaluate and disseminate broadly the research on the health impacts of efforts to reduce financial burdens associated with the treatment of hypertension.

The use of community health workers to support the care of individuals with hypertension has been identified as a promising strategy. Community health workers have contributed to greater medication adherence among individuals with hypertension and have been shown to play an important role in linking diverse communities to the health care system and navigating that system.

5.5 The committee recommends that the Division for Heart Disease and Stroke Prevention work with state partners to leverage opportunities to ensure that existing community health worker programs include a focus on the prevention and control of hypertension. In the absence of such programs, the division should work with state partners to develop programs of community health workers who would be deployed in high-risk communities to help support healthy living strategies that include a focus on hypertension.

REFERENCES

Adams, A. S., S. B. Soumerai, and D. Ross-Degnan. 2001a. The case for a Medicare drug coverage benefit: A critical review of the empirical evidence. *Annual Review of Public Health* 22:49-61.

———. 2001b. Use of antihypertensive drugs by Medicare enrollees: Does type of drug coverage matter? *Health Affairs* 20(1):276-286.

Ahluwalia, J. S., S. E. McNagny, and K. J. Rask. 1997. Correlates of controlled hypertension in indigent, inner-city hypertensive patients. *Journal of General Internal Medicine* 12(1):7-14.

AHRQ (Agency for Healthcare Research and Quality). 2004. *Closing the quality gap: A critical analysis of hypertension care strategies.* http://www.ahrq.gov/qual/hypertengap.htm (accessed October 28, 2009).

Aldana, S. G. 2001. Financial impact of health promotion programs: A comprehensive review of the literature. *American Journal of Health Promotion* 15(5):296-320.

AMA (American Medical Association). 2006. *Hypertension (HTN): Algorithm for measures calculation—EHRS.* http://www.ama-assn.org/ama1/pub/upload/mm/370/htnanalyticnarr 307_7.pdf (accessed February 5, 2010).

American College of Sports Medicine. 2009. *ACSM's worksite health handbook-2nd edition: A guide to building healthy and productive companies.* Edited by N. P. Pronk. Champaign, IL: American College of Sports Medicine.

Anis, A. H., D. P. Guh, D. Lacaille, C. A. Marra, A. A. Rashidi, X. Li, and J. M. Esdaile. 2005. When patients have to pay a share of drug costs: Effects on frequency of physician visits, hospital admissions and filling of prescriptions. *Canadian Medical Association Journal* 173(11):1335-1340.

Artz, M. B., R. S. Hadsall, and S. W. Schondelmeyer. 2002. Impact of generosity level of outpatient prescription drug coverage on prescription drug events and expenditure among older persons. *American Journal of Public Health* 92(8):1257-1263.

Austvoll-Dahlgren, A., M. Aaserud, G. Vist, C. Ramsay, A. D. Oxman, H. Sturm, J. P. Kosters, and A. Vernby. 2008. Pharmaceutical policies: Effects of cap and co-payment on rational drug use. *Cochrane Database of Systematic Reviews* (1).

Ayanian, J. Z., J. S. Weissman, E. C. Schneider, J. A. Ginsburg, and A. M. Zaslavsky. 2000. Unmet health needs of uninsured adults in the United States. *Journal of the American Medical Association* 284(16):2061-2069.

Berlowitz, D. R., A. S. Ash, E. C. Hickey, R. H. Friedman, M. Glickman, B. Kader, and M. A. Moskowitz. 1998. Inadequate management of blood pressure in a hypertensive population. *New England Journal of Medicine* 339(27):1957-1963.

Blais, L., J. M. Boucher, J. Couture, E. Rahme, and J. LeLorier. 2001. Impact of a cost-sharing drug insurance plan on drug utilization among older people. *Journal of the American Geriatrics Society* 49(4):410-414.

Blustein, J. 2000. Drug coverage and drug purchases by Medicare beneficiaries with hypertension. *Health Affairs* 19(2):219-230.

Bokhour, B. G., D. R. Berlowitz, J. A. Long, and N. R. Kressin. 2006. How do providers assess antihypertensive medication adherence in medical encounters? *Journal of General Internal Medicine* 21(6):577-583.

Bosworth, H. B., M. K. Olsen, P. Gentry, M. Orr, T. Dudley, F. McCant, and E. Z. Oddone. 2005. Nurse administered telephone intervention for blood pressure control: A patient-tailored multifactorial intervention. *Patient Education and Counseling* 57(1):5-14.

Bray, G. A., W. M. Vollmer, F. M. Sacks, E. Obarzanek, L. P. Svetkey, and L. J. Appel. 2004. A further subgroup analysis of the effects of the DASH diet and three dietary sodium levels on blood pressure: Results of the DASH-sodium trial. *American Journal of Cardiology* 94(2):222-227.

Brook, R. H., J. E. Ware, W. H. Rogers, E. B. Keeler, A. R. Davies, C. A. Donald, G. A. Goldberg, K. N. Lohr, P. C. Masthay, and J. P. Newhouse. 1983. Does free care improve adults health—results from a randomized controlled trial. *New England Journal of Medicine* 309(23):1426-1434.

Brownstein, J. N., L. R. Bone, C. R. Dennison, M. N. Hill, M. T. Kim, and D. M. Levine. 2005. Community health workers as interventionists in the prevention and control of heart disease and stroke. *American Journal of Preventive Medicine* 29(5 Suppl 1):128-133.

Brownstein, J. N., F. M. Chowdhury, S. L. Norris, T. Horsley, L. Jack Jr, X. Zhang, and D. Satterfield. 2007. Effectiveness of community health workers in the care of people with hypertension. *American Journal of Preventive Medicine* 32(5):435-447.

Capozza, K. 2008. *First-dollar coverage for chronic disease care: Can it save money and improve patient outcomes?* Berkeley, CA: UC Berkeley Labor Center.

CDC (Centers for Disease Control and Prevention). 1994. Health objectives for the nation: Adults taking action to control their blood pressure—United States, 1990. *Morbidity and Mortality Weekly Report* 43(28):509-511.

———. 2008a. *The community health worker's sourcebook: A training manual for preventing heart disease and stroke.* Atlanta, GA: Division for Heart Disease and Stroke Prevention.

———. 2008b. *Successful business strategies to prevent heart disease and stroke.* Atlanta, GA: Centers for Disease Control and Prevention.

———. 2009. *The National Business Group on Health.* http://www.cdc.gov/Partners/Business/NBGH.html (accessed November 4, 2009).

CDC and NBGH (National Business Group on Health). 2006. *A Purchaser's Guide to Clinical Preventive Services: Moving Science into Coverage.* Washington, DC: National Business Group on Health.

Chernew, M. E., A. B. Rosen, and A. M. Fendrick. 2007. Value-based insurance design. *Health Affairs* 26(2):w195-w203.

Chiong, J. R. 2008. Controlling hypertension from a public health perspective. *International Journal of Cardiology* 127(2):151-156.

Chockalingam, A., M. Bacher, N. Campbell, H. Cutler, A. Drover, R. Feldman, G. Fodor, J. Irvine, V. Ramsden, R. Thivierge, and G. Tremblay. 1998. Adherence to management of high blood pressure: Recommendations of the Canadian coalition for high blood pressure prevention and control. *Canadian Journal of Public Health* (Revue Canadienne de Sante Publique) 89(5):I5-I11.

Clark, L. T. 1991. Improving compliance and increasing control of hypertension: Needs of special hypertensive populations. *American Heart Journal* 121(2 Pt 2):664-669.

Col, N., J. E. Fanale, and P. Kronholm. 1990. The role of medication noncompliance and adverse drug reactions in hospitalizations of the elderly. *Archives of Internal Medicine* 150(4):841-845.

Cox, E. R., C. Jernigan, S. J. Coons, and J. L. Draugalis. 2001. Medicare beneficiaries' management of capped prescription benefits. *Medical Care* 39(3):296-301.

Eddy, D. M., L. G. Pawlson, D. Schaaf, B. Peskin, A. Shcheprov, J. Dziuba, J. Bowman, and B. Eng. 2008. The potential effects of HEDIS performance measures on the quality of care. *Health Affairs* 27(5):1429-1441.

Ekpo, E. B., I. U. Shah, M. U. Fernando, and A. D. White. 1993. Isolated systolic hypertension in the elderly: Survey of practitioners' attitude and management. *Gerontology* 39(4):207-214.

Elliott, W. J. 2003. Optimizing medication adherence in older persons with hypertension. *International Urology and Nephrology* 35(4):557-562.

Fairman, K. A., B. R. Motheral, and R. R. Henderson. 2003. Retrospective, long-term follow-up study of the effect of a three-tier prescription drug copayment system on pharmaceutical and other medical utilization and costs. *Clinical Therapeutics* 25(12):3147-3161; discussion 3144-3146.

Fihn, S. D., and J. B. Wicher. 1988. Withdrawing routine outpatient medical services: Effects on access and health. *Journal of General Internal Medicine* 3(4):356-362.

Franklin, S. S., M. J. Jacobs, N. D. Wong, G. J. L'Italien, and P. Lapuerta. 2001. Predominance of isolated systolic hypertension among middle-aged and elderly US hypertensives: Analysis based on National Health and Nutrition Examination Survey (NHANES) III. *Hypertension* 37(3):869-874.

Gallup, G., and H. E. Cotugno. 1986. Preferences and practices of Americans and their physicians in antihypertensive therapy. *American Journal of Medicine* 81(6C):20-24.

Goetzel, R. Z., and R. J. Ozminkowski. 2008. The health and cost benefits of work site health-promotion programs. *Annual Review of Public Health* 29:303-323.

Goetzel, R. Z., D. Shechter, R. J. Ozminkowski, P. F. Marmet, M. J. Tabrizi, and E. C. Roemer. 2007. Promising practices in employer health and productivity management efforts: Findings from a benchmarking study. *Journal of Occupational and Environmental Medicine* 49(2):111-130.

Goldman, D. P., G. F. Joyce, J. J. Escarce, J. E. Pace, M. D. Solomon, M. Laouri, P. B. Landsman, and S. M. Teutsch. 2004. Pharmacy benefits and the use of drugs by the chronically ill. *Journal of the American Medical Association* 291(19):2344-2350.

Goldman, D. P., G. F. Joyce, and Y. Zheng. 2007. Prescription drug cost sharing: Associations with medication and medical utilization and spending and health. *Journal of the American Medical Association* 298(1):61-69.

Gu, Q., V. L. Burt, R. Paulose-Ram, S. Yoon, and R. F. Gillum. 2008. High blood pressure and cardiovascular disease mortality risk among U.S. adults: The Third National Health and Nutrition Examination Survey Mortality Follow-up study. *Annals of Epidemiology* 18(4):302-309.

Guide to Community Preventive Services. 2009. *Assessment of health risks with feedback to change employees' health.* www.thecommunityguide.org/worksite/ahrf.html (accessed November 4, 2009).

Halm, J., and E. Amoako. 2008. Physical activity recommendation for hypertension man-
    agement: Does healthcare provider advice make a difference? *Ethnicity and Disease*
    18(3):278-282.
Harmon, G., J. Lefante, and M. Krousel-Wood. 2006. Overcoming barriers: The role of pro-
    viders in improving patient adhereence to antihypertensive medications. *Current Opinion
    in Cardiology* 21(4):310-315.
Harris, B. L., A. Stergachis, and L. D. Ried. 1990. The effect of drug co-payments on utiliza-
    tion and cost of pharmaceuticals in a health maintenance organization. *Medical Care*
    28(10):907-917.
He, J., P. Muntner, J. Chen, E. J. Roccella, R. H. Streiffer, and P. K. Whelton. 2002. Factors
    associated with hypertension control in the general population of the United States.
    Archives of Internal Medicine 162(9):1051-1058.
HRSA (Health Resources and Services Administration). 2007. *Community health worker
    national workforce study*: U.S. Department of Health and Human Services.
Hsu, J., M. Price, J. Huang, R. Brand, V. Fung, R. Hui, B. Fireman, J. P. Newhouse, and J. V.
    Selby. 2006. Unintended consequences of caps on Medicare drug benefits. *New England
    Journal of Medicine* 354(22):2349-2359.
Huskamp, H. A., P. A. Deverka, A. M. Epstein, R. S. Epstein, K. A. McGuigan, and R. G.
    Frank. 2003. The effect of incentive-based formularies on prescription-drug utilization
    and spending. *New England Journal of Medicine* 349(23):2224-2232.
Hyman, D. J., and V. N. Pavlik. 2000. Self-reported hypertension treatment practices among
    primary care physicians—blood pressure thresholds, drug choices, and the role of guide-
    lines and evidence-based medicine. *Archives of Internal Medicine* 160(15):2281-2286.
————. 2001. Characteristics of patients with uncontrolled hypertension in the United States.
    [see comment] [erratum appears in 2002 *New England Journal of Medicine* 346(7):544].
    New England Journal of Medicine 345(7):479-486.
Hyman, D. J., V. N. Pavlik, and C. Vallbona. 2000. Physician role in lack of awareness and
    control of hypertension. *Journal of Clinical Hypertension (Greenwich)* 2(5):324-330.
IOM (Institute of Medicine). 2000. *To err is human: Building a safer health system*. Washing-
    ton, DC: National Academy Press.
————. 2001a. *Coverage matters: Insurance and health care*. Washington, DC: National
    Academy Press.
————. 2001b. *Crossing the quality chasm: A new health system for the 21st century*. Wash-
    ington, DC: National Academy Press.
————. 2002a. *Care without coverage: Too little, too late*. Washington, DC: The National
    Academies Press.
————. 2002b. *Health insurance is a family matter*. Washington, DC: The National Acad-
    emies Press.
————. 2003a. *The future of public health in the 21st century*. Washington, DC: The National
    Academies Press.
————. 2003b. *Hidden costs, value lost: Uninsurance in America*. Washington, DC: The
    National Academies Press.
————. 2003c. *Priority areas for national action: Transforming health care quality*. Washing-
    ton, DC: The National Academies Press.
————. 2003d. *A shared destiny: Community effects of uninsurance*. Washington, DC: The
    National Academies Press.
————. 2003e. *Unequal treatment: Confronting racial and ethnic disparities in health care*.
    Washington DC: The National Academies Press.
————. 2004. *Insuring America's health: Principles and recommendations*. Washington, DC:
    The National Academies Press.

Izzo, J. L., Jr., D. Levy, and H. R. Black. 2000. Clinical advisory statement. Importance of systolic blood pressure in older Americans. *Hypertension* 35(5):1021-1024.

Johnson, R. E., M. J. Goodman, M. C. Hornbrook, and M. B. Eldredge. 1997a. The effect of increased prescription drug cost-sharing on medical care utilization and expenses of elderly health maintenance organization members. *Medical Care* 35(11):1119-1131.

———. 1997b. The impact of increasing patient prescription drug cost sharing on therapeutic classes of drugs received and on the health status of elderly HMO members. *Health Services Research* 32(1):103-122.

Kamal-Bahl, S., and B. Briesacher. 2004. How do incentive-based formularies influence drug selection and spending for hypertension? *Health Affairs* 23(1):227-236.

Keeler, E. B., R. H. Brook, G. A. Goldberg, C. J. Kamberg, and J. P. Newhouse. 1985. How free care reduced hypertension in the Health Insurance Experiment. *Journal of the American Medical Association* 254(14):1926-1931.

Keeler, E. B., E. M. Sloss, R. H. Brook, B. H. Operskalski, G. A. Goldberg, and J. P. Newhouse. 1987. Effects of cost sharing on physiological health, health practices, and worry. *Health Services Research* 22(3):279-306.

Koffman, M., M. Molloy, L. Agin, and L. Sokler. 2005. *Reducing the risk of heart disease and stroke: A six-step guide for employers.* Atlanta, GA: Centers for Disease Control and Prevention, U.S. Department of Health and Human Services.

Kokkinos, P. F., P. Narayan, J. A. Colleran, A. Pittaras, A. Notargiacomo, D. Reda, and V. Papademetriou. 1995. Effects of regular exercise on blood-pressure and left-ventricular hypertrophy in African-American men with severe hypertension. *New England Journal of Medicine* 333(22):1462-1467.

Kotchen, J. M., B. Shakoor-Abdullah, W. E. Walker, T. H. Chelius, R. G. Hoffmann, and T. A. Kotchen. 1998. Hypertension control and access to medical care in the inner city. *American Journal of Public Health* 88(11):1696-1699.

Krousel-Wood, M., A. Hyre, P. Muntner, and D. Morisky. 2005. Methods to improve medication adherence in patients with hypertension: Current status and future directions. *Current Opinion in Cardiology* 20(4):296-300.

Landsman, P. B., W. Yu, X. Liu, S. M. Teutsch, and M. L. Berger. 2005. Impact of 3-tier pharmacy benefit design and increased consumer cost-sharing on drug utilization. *American Journal of Managed Care* 11(10):621-628.

Lexchin, J., and P. Grootendorst. 2004. Effects of prescription drug user fees on drug and health services use and on health status in vulnerable populations: A systematic review of the evidence. *International Journal of Health Services* 34(1):101-122.

Lloyd-Jones, D. M., J. C. Evans, M. G. Larson, C. J. O'Donnell, E. J. Roccella, and D. Levy. 2000. Differential control of systolic and diastolic blood pressure: Factors associated with lack of blood pressure control in the community. *Hypertension* 36(4):594-599.

Lloyd-Jones, D. M., J. C. Evans, M. G. Larson, and D. Levy. 2002. Treatment and control of hypertension in the community: A prospective analysis. *Hypertension* 40(5):640-646.

Lohr, K. N., R. H. Brook, C. J. Kamberg, G. A. Goldberg, A. Leibowitz, J. Keesey, D. Reboussin, and J. P. Newhouse. 1986. Use of medical care in the Rand Health Insurance Experiment. Diagnosis- and service-specific analyses in a randomized controlled trial. *Medical Care* 24(9 Suppl):S1-S87.

Lopes, A. A., S. A. James, F. K. Port, A. O. Ojo, L. Y. Agodoa, and K. A. Jamerson. 2003. Meeting the challenge to improve the treatment of hypertension in blacks. *Journal of Clinical Hypertension (Greenwich)* 5(6):393-401.

Lurie, N., N. B. Ward, M. F. Shapiro, and R. H. Brook. 1984. Termination from Medi-Cal—does it affect health? *New England Journal of Medicine* 311(7):480-484.

Lurie, N., N. B. Ward, M. F. Shapiro, C. Gallego, R. Vaghaiwalla, and R. H. Brook. 1986. Termination of Medi-Cal benefits. A follow-up study one year later. *New England Journal of Medicine* 314(19):1266-1268.

Maciosek, M. V., A. B. Coffield, N. M. Edwards, T. J. Flottemesch, M. J. Goodman, and L. I. Solberg. 2006. Priorities among effective clinical preventive services: Results of a systematic review and analysis. *American Journal of Preventive Medicine* 31(1):52-61.

Maronde, R. F., L. S. Chan, F. J. Larsen, L. R. Strandberg, M. F. Laventurier, and S. R. Sullivan. 1989. Underutilization of antihypertensive drugs and associated hospitalization. *Medical Care* 27(12):1159-1166.

McCombs, J. S., M. B. Nichol, C. M. Newman, and D. A. Sclar. 1994. The costs of interrupting antihypertensive drug therapy in a Medicaid population. *Medical Care* 32(3):214-226.

Mellen, P. B., S. L. Palla, D. C. Goff Jr., and D. E. Bonds. 2004. Prevalence of nutrition and exercise counseling for patients with hypertension. *Journal of General Internal Medicine* 19(9):917-924.

Mojtabai, R., and M. Olfson. 2003. Medication costs, adherence, and health outcomes among Medicare beneficiaries. *Health Affairs* 22(4):220-229.

Motheral, B., and K. A. Fairman. 2001. Effect of a three-tier prescription copay on pharmaceutical and other medical utilization. *Medical Care* 39(12):1293-1304.

Motheral, B. R., and R. Henderson. 1999a. The effect of a closed formulary on prescription drug use and costs. *Inquiry-the Journal of Health Care Organization Provision and Financing* 36(4):481-491.

———. 1999b. The effect of a copay increase on pharmaceutical utilization, expenditures, and treatment continuation. *American Journal of Managed Care* 5(11):1383-1394.

Moy, E., B. A. Bartman, and M. R. Weir. 1995. Access to hypertensive care. Effects of income, insurance, and source of care. *Archives of Internal Medicine* 155(14):1497-1502.

Nair, K. V., P. Wolfe, R. J. Valuck, M. M. McCollum, J. M. Ganther, and S. J. Lewis. 2003. Effects of a 3-tier pharmacy benefit design on the prescription purchasing behavior of individuals with chronic disease. *Journal of Managed Care Pharmacy* 9(2):123-133.

NCQA (National Committee for Quality Assurance). 2009. *The state of health care quality*. Washington, DC: National Committee for Quality Assurance.

NHLBI (National Heart, Lung, and Blood Institute). 2006a. *Honoring the gift of heart health: A heart health educator's manual for Alaska Natives*. Bethesda, MD: U.S. Department of Health and Human Services.

NHLBI. 2006b. *Honoring the gift of heart health: A heart health educator's manual for American Indians*. Bethesda, MD: U.S. Department of Health and Human Services.

NHLBI. 2007. *With every heartbeat is life: A community health worker's manual for African Americans*. Bethesda, MD: U.S. Department of Health and Human Services.

NHLBI. 2008a. *Healthy heart, healthy family: A community health worker's manual for the Filipino community*. Bethesda, MD: U.S. Department of Health and Human Services.

NHLBI. 2008b. *Your heart, your life: A community health worker's manual for the Hispanic community*. Bethesda, MD: U.S. Department of Health and Human Services.

Okonofua, E. C., K. N. Simpson, A. Jesri, S. U. Rehman, V. L. Durkalski, and B. M. Egan. 2006. Therapeutic inertia is an impediment to achieving the Healthy People 2010 blood pressure control goals. *Hypertension* 47(3):345-351.

Oliveria, S. A., P. Lapuerta, B. D. McCarthy, G. J. L'Italien, D. R. Berlowitz, and S. M. Asch. 2002. Physician-related barriers to the effective management of uncontrolled hypertension. *Archives of Internal Medicine* 162(4):413-420.

Partnership for Prevention. 2001. *Healthy workforce 2010: An essential health promotion sourcebook for employers, large and small*. Washington, DC: Partnership for Prevention.

————. 2006. *Priorities for America's health: Capitalizing on life-saving, cost-effective preventive services.* Washington, DC: Partnership for Prevention.

Pavlik, V. N., D. J. Hyman, C. Vallbona, C. Toronjo, and K. Louis. 1997. Hypertension awareness and control in an inner-city African-American sample. *Journal of Human Hypertension* 11(5):277-283.

Piette, J. D., M. Heisler, and T. H. Wagner. 2004. Cost-related medication underuse among chronically ill adults: The treatments people forgo, how often, and who is at risk. *American Journal of Public Health* 94(10):1782-1787.

Poirier, S., and J. LeLorier. 1998. The effect of a $2 co-payment on prescription refill rates of Quebec elderly and its relationship to socioeconomic status. *Canadian Pharmacy Journal* 131(1):30-34.

RAND. 2006. *The first national report card on quality of health care in America.* Santa Monica, CA: RAND Corporation.

Reeder, C. E., and A. A. Nelson. 1985. The differential impact of copayment on drug use in a Medicaid population. *Inquiry* 22(4):396-403.

Rogowski, J., L. A. Lillard, and R. Kington. 1997. The financial burden of prescription drug use among elderly persons. *Gerontologist* 37(4):475-482.

Schneeweiss, S., S. B. Soumerai, R. J. Glynn, M. Maclure, C. Dormuth, and A. M. Walker. 2002a. Impact of reference-based pricing for angiotensin-converting enzyme inhibitors on drug utilization. *Canadian Medical Association Journal* 166(6):737-745.

Schneeweiss, S., A. M. Walker, R. J. Glynn, M. Maclure, C. Dormuth, and S. B. Soumerai. 2002b. Outcomes of reference pricing for angiotensin-converting-enzyme inhibitors. *New England Journal of Medicine* 346(11):822-829.

Schulz, R. M., E. W. Lingle, S. J. Chubon, and M. A. Coster-Schulz. 1995. Drug use behavior under the constraints of a Medicaid prescription cap. *Clinical Therapeutics* 17(2):330-340.

Shea, S., D. Misra, M. H. Ehrlich, L. Field, and C. K. Francis. 1992a. Correlates of nonadherence to hypertension treatment in an inner-city minority population. *American Journal of Public Health* 82(12):1607-1612.

————. 1992b. Predisposing factors for severe, uncontrolled hypertension in an inner-city minority population. *New England Journal of Medicine* 327(11):776-781.

SHEP Cooperative Research Group. 1991. Prevention of stroke by antihypertensive drug treatment in older persons with isolated systolic hypertension. Final results of the Systolic Hypertension in the Elderly Program (SHEP). SHEP cooperative research group. *Journal of the American Medical Association* 265(24):3255-3264.

Shrank, W. H., T. Hoang, S. L. Ettner, P. A. Glassman, K. Nair, D. DeLapp, J. Dirstine, J. Avorn, and S. M. Asch. 2006. The implications of choice: Prescribing generic or preferred pharmaceuticals improves medication adherence for chronic conditions. *Archives of Internal Medicine* 166(3):332-337.

Shulman, N. B., B. Martinez, D. Brogan, A. A. Carr, and C. G. Miles. 1986. Financial cost as an obstacle to hypertension therapy. *American Journal of Public Health* 76(9):1105-1108.

Solomon, M. D., D. P. Goldman, G. F. Joyce, and J. J. Escarce. 2009. Cost sharing and the initiation of drug therapy for the chronically ill. *Archives of Internal Medicine* 169(8):740-748; discussion 748-749.

Soumerai, S. B., D. Ross-Degnan, J. Avorn, T. McLaughlin, and I. Choodnovskiy. 1991. Effects of Medicaid drug-payment limits on admission to hospitals and nursing homes. *New England Journal of Medicine* 325(15):1072-1077.

Soumerai, S. B., T. J. Mclaughlin, D. Rossdegnan, C. S. Casteris, and P. Bollini. 1994. Effects of limiting Medicaid drug-reimbursement benefits on the use of psychotropic agents and acute mental-health-services by patients with schizophrenia. *New England Journal of Medicine* 331(10):650-655.

Steinman, M. A., L. P. Sands, and K. E. Covinsky. 2001. Self-restriction of medications due to cost in seniors without prescription coverage. *Journal of General Internal Medicine* 16(12):793-799.

Steinman, M. A., M. A. Fischer, M. G. Shlipak, H. B. Bosworth, E. Z. Oddone, B. B. Hoffman, and M. K. Goldstein. 2004. Clinician awareness of adherence to hypertension guidelines. *American Journal of Medicine* 117(10):747-754.

Stockwell, D. H., S. Madhavan, H. Cohen, G. Gibson, and M. H. Alderman. 1994. The determinants of hypertension awareness, treatment, and control in an insured population. *American Journal of Public Health* 84(11):1768-1774.

Stuart, B., and J. Grana. 1998. Ability to pay and the decision to medicate. *Medical Care* 36(2):202-211.

Svetkey, L. P., D. Simons-Morton, W. M. Vollmer, L. J. Appel, P. R. Conlin, D. H. Ryan, J. Ard, and B. M. Kennedy. 1999. Effects of dietary patterns on blood pressure: Subgroup analysis of the Dietary Approaches to Stop Hypertension (DASH) randomized clinical trial. *Archives of Internal Medicine* 159(3):285-293.

Taira, D. A., K. S. Wong, F. Frech-Tamas, and R. S. Chung. 2006. Copayment level and compliance with antihypertensive medication: Analysis and policy implications for managed care. *American Journal of Managed Care* 12(11):678-683.

Tamblyn, R., R. Laprise, J. A. Hanley, M. Abrahamowicz, S. Scott, N. Mayo, J. Hurley, R. Grad, E. Latimer, R. Perreault, P. McLeod, A. Huang, P. Larochelle, and L. Mallet. 2001. Adverse events associated with prescription drug cost-sharing among poor and elderly persons. *Journal of the American Medical Association* 285(4):421-429.

Tseng, C. W., R. H. Brook, E. Keeler, W. N. Steers, and C. M. Mangione. 2004. Cost-lowering strategies used by Medicare beneficiaries who exceed drug benefit caps and have a gap in drug coverage. *Journal of the American Medical Association* 292(8):952-960.

Vollmer, W. M., L. P. Svetkey, L. J. Appel, E. Obarzanek, P. Reams, B. Kennedy, K. Aicher, J. Charleston, P. R. Conlin, M. Evans, D. Harsha, and S. Hertert. 1998. Recruitment and retention of minority participants in the DASH controlled feeding trial. DASH Collaborative Research Group. Dietary Approaches to Stop Hypertension. *Ethnicity and Disease* 8(2):198-208.

Weissman, J. S., C. Gatsonis, and A. M. Epstein. 1992. Rates of avoidable hospitalization by insurance status in Massachusetts and Maryland. *Journal of the American Medical Association* 268(17):2388-2394.

Wilson, J., K. Axelsen, and S. Tang. 2005. Medicaid prescription drug access restrictions: Exploring the effect on patient persistence with hypertension medications. *American Journal of Managed Care* 11(Spec No):SP27-SP34.

Witmer, A., S. D. Seifer, L. Finocchio, J. Leslie, and E. H. O'Neil. 1995. Community health workers: Integral members of the health care work force. *American Journal of Public Health* 85(8 Pt 1):1055-1058.

Woolhandler, S., and D. U. Himmelstein. 1988. Reverse targeting of preventive care due to lack of health insurance. *Journal of the American Medical Association* 259(19):2872-2874.

Wright, J. T., Jr., G. Bakris, T. Greene, L. Y. Agodoa, L. J. Appel, J. Charleston, D. Cheek, J. G. Douglas-Baltimore, J. Gassman, R. Glassock, L. Hebert, K. Jamerson, J. Lewis, R. A. Phillips, R. D. Toto, J. P. Middleton, S., and G. Rostand, for the African American Study of Kidney Disease and Hypertension Study Group. 2002. Effect of blood pressure lowering and antihypertensive drug class on progression of hypertensive kidney disease: Results from the AASK trial. [see comment] [erratum appears in 2006 *Journal of the American Medical Association* 295(23):2726]. *Journal of the American Medical Association* 288(19):2421-2431.

6

Implementing a Population-Based Policy and Systems Approach to the Prevention and Control of Hypertension

Hypertension is highly prevalent in adults, endemic in the elderly, a major contributor to cardiovascular mortality and disability, costly to our society, and a substantial contributor to health disparities in the United States. Hypertension is also simple to diagnose, relatively inexpensive to treat, and more importantly, is highly preventable through lifestyle interventions.

Despite these facts, surprisingly and unfortunately, hypertension does not receive a level of attention and funding commensurate with its associated health burden and consequences, and the public health approach to addressing hypertension in this decade has suffered. The early national attention to hypertension of the 1970s (National High Blood Pressure Education Program) has diminished, and the focus on prevention and early detection has shifted toward pharmacologic treatment. This lack of attention is exacerbated, in part, because hypertension as a condition sits between more primary risk factors such as diet and physical activity and medical disease states such as cardiovascular and cerebrovascular disease, with consequent ambiguity in leadership and diffusion of responsibility between public health and medical care. From the perspective of those affected, hypertension is easy to neglect. It is not an apparent risk factor such as smoking or obesity, and, for the majority of individuals, it causes no symptoms. Thus there has been little "ownership" for the prevention of hypertension.

The Centers for Disease Control and Prevention (CDC), through the Division for Heart Disease and Stroke Prevention (DHDSP), has leveraged its broader cardiovascular disease prevention and control programmatic efforts to address hypertension primarily through its state heart disease and stroke prevention programs. Many of these efforts are described in Chapter 3 and throughout other chapters. Objectively, however, there are two significant problems with the current status and direction of hypertension prevention and control activities:

- Hypertension is only one component of a larger cardiovascular disease prevention program that has more of a medical care rather than a population-based prevention focus.
- The CDC's cardiovascular disease program in general, and the hypertension program in particular, are dramatically under funded relative to the preventable burden of disease and the strategy and action plan that have been developed. Despite the magnitude of hypertension-associated morbidity and mortality and costs to the health care system ($73 billion annually), the current resources available for hypertension prevention and control at the CDC are surprisingly limited ($54 million for all cardiovascular and stroke activities in 2009).

This current economic reality limiting the absolute amount of resources available to the CDC must drive short-term programmatic priorities towards approaches that are not only cost-effective but also low in absolute cost. Compared with interventions directed toward individuals, interventions directed toward policy, systems, and environmental changes in populations are more likely to be realistic and effective in the current resource-constrained environment. The committee believes that the DHDSP should focus its priorities on approaches that cater to the strength of the public health system—population-based policy and systems approaches rather than individual health care-based approaches. Any investments in the health care sector should be policy- and systems-based and should leverage health care system resources.

The committee has recommended a number of high-priority strategies to prevent and control hypertension to the DHDSP throughout Chapters 4 and 5. The recommendations embody a population-based policy and systems approach grounded in the principles of measurement, system change, and accountability. In brief, the recommendations seek to:

- Shift the balance of the DHDSP's hypertension priorities from individual-based strategies to population-based strategies to:
  o strengthen collaboration among CDC units (and their partners) to ensure that hypertension is included as a dimension of other population-based activities around healthy lifestyle improvement, particularly greater consumption of potassium-rich

fruits and vegetables, increased physical activity, and weight management
  o strengthen CDC's leadership in monitoring and reducing sodium intake in the American diet to meet current dietary guidelines
  o improve the surveillance and reporting of hypertension to better characterize general trends and trends among subgroups of the population
- Promote policy and *system* change approaches to:
  o improve the quality of care provided to individuals by assuring that individuals who should be in treatment are in treatment and receive care that is consistent with current treatment guidelines
    ♦ increase the importance of treating systolic hypertension, especially among the elderly
  o remove economic barriers to effective antihypertensive medications
  o provide community-based support for individuals with hypertension through community health workers who are trained in dietary and physical activity counseling.

The committee, through these recommendations, underscores the importance of policy, systems, and environmental change interventions as fundamental to preventing and controlling hypertension. Clearly, this approach cannot be limited to the CDC DHDSP but must also extend to state and local health departments and other partners responsible for implementing these interventions. Successfully implementing a population-based policy and systems approach at all levels will depend on the resources available and systems of accountability to ensure that resources are appropriately aligned and outcomes are achieved. In the next section the committee makes recommendations for state and local health jurisdictions, including necessary resources and accountability measures to support the recommended population-based policy and systems approach to preventing and controlling hypertension.

RECOMMENDATIONS FOR STATE AND LOCAL HEALTH JURISDICTIONS

State and local governments have specific roles and responsibilities for protecting, preserving, and promoting the public's health. They fulfill their responsibility through many activities including monitoring injury and disease in the population through surveillance systems; providing a broad array of population-wide prevention services; and helping to assure access to high-quality health care services for poor and vulnerable populations. They also engage in a broad array of regulatory activities, and they oversee the quality of health care provided in the public and private sectors (IOM, 2002). State and local public health agencies can act on the most upstream level of determinants of health. Action at this level may help to shift norms and values and lead to policies that promote health (for example, state and local tobacco policies). Thus, as with federal public health agencies, state and local public health agencies are uniquely skilled in population-based interventions and in general have more experience in these interventions than in interventions that directly provide health care to individuals.

The committee views population-based approaches to prevent and control hypertension at the state and local level to be consistent with the broad mandates of state and local public health jurisdictions (SLHJs).

6.1 The Committee recommends that state and local public health jurisdictions give priority to population-based approaches over individual-based approaches to prevent and control hypertension.

Population-based policy and systems interventions for hypertension prevention and control are arguably the most important and relevant component of hypertension programming for SLHJs. By their nature, many elements of hypertension prevention fit neatly into current SLHJs' programs for healthy eating, active living, and obesity prevention (IOM, 2007, 2009). As such, population approaches to hypertension should be integrated into these existing efforts rather than re-created as separate, stand alone programs. At the same time, these existing programs may need adjustment and expansion. For example, the high prevalence of hypertension in older populations and other population subgroups (African Americans) should lead SLHJs to assess and, if necessary, modify these programs to assure they are relevant and accessible to older and higher-risk populations.

6.2 The committee recommends that state and local public health jurisdictions integrate hypertension prevention and control in programmatic efforts to effect system, environmental, and policy changes that will support healthy eating, active living, and obesity prevention. Existing and new programmatic efforts should be assessed to ensure they are aligned with populations most likely to be affected by hypertension such as older populations, which are often not the target of these programs.

A major risk factor for hypertension—excess sodium consumption in the diet—currently is not targeted by most SLHJs and is a new, important target for public health action. Strategies for sodium reduction will be further refined in an upcoming IOM report by the Committee on Strategies to Reduce Sodium Intake (slated to be released in early 2010) but may include:

> public education to increase awareness of the importance of reduced sodium in the diet and the salt content of foods; modifying sodium policies in food programs under SLHJs jurisdiction; voluntary or regulatory measures to reduce sodium levels in processed foods and foods prepared in institutions such as schools and worksites.

Actions to reduce sodium levels in food products have been initiated by other countries including the United Kingdom (UK) and are showing some impact. The UK Food Standards Agency published voluntary salt reduction targets in March 2006 to lower population salt intake from 9.5 g (baseline in 2000-2001) to 6 g per day. Since that time, the agency has been working with health departments, directorates and stakeholders, and industry to reduce salt consumption in the UK. A recent progress review indicated that many companies that produce processed foods have programs in place to reduce salt and have met targets for specific categories. Urinary analysis results taken in January and May 2008 indicate that overall salt reduction initiatives (public awareness, industry activities, and others) have decreased average salt intake to 8.6 g based on dietary sodium in 24-hour urine samples (National Centre for Social Research, 2008).

In the United States, cities, states, and national health organizations are taking steps to reduce population salt intake; the National Salt Reduction Initiative (NSRI), coordinated by the New York City (NYC) Health Department, has led the way. The NSRI's strategy includes working with the food industry to set sodium reduction targets for their products that are substantive, achievable, gradual, measurable, and voluntary, with the goal of reducing population sodium intake by 20 percent over 5 years. The process for implementing the strategy includes meeting with food industry leaders to discuss sodium reduction, working with packaged food manufacturers and restaurants to set voluntary sodium targets by food category, implementing targets and timelines to reduce salt, and monitoring the salt reduction process through the creation of restaurant and packaged food nutrition databases. Across the country 26 state and local public health agencies and 17 professional associations and organizations have coalesced into the NSRI (The City of New York, 2009).

6.3 The committee recommends that all state and local public health jurisdictions immediately begin to consider developing a portfolio of dietary sodium reduction strategies that make the most sense for early action in their jurisdictions.

Reliable, ongoing measurement of a public health problem is essential to its effective control. Blood pressure is relatively simple to measure, however, access to and use of hypertension measures at the SLHJs level has proven difficult. The primary national data source for population estimates of hypertension—National Health and Nutrition Examination Survey (NHANES)—is not designed to produce accurate state or local estimates. This shortcoming is a major one, as there is likely substantial variation across regions not only in prevalence but also in the proportions of the hypertensive population not diagnosed, diagnosed but not under treatment, and under treatment but not controlled. The primary risk factor surveillance system used by SLHJs, the Behavioral Risk Factor Surveillance System, is limited because it relies on self-report rather than objective measurement, and it provides no information on the extent and characteristics of undiagnosed hypertension. In short, SLHJs do not have the basic data that would be most useful in assessing need and driving local policy interventions; this lack of data may contribute to the relative inattention to hypertension by SLHJs to date.

Hypertension provides one of the most compelling conditions justifying the creation of a state and local NHANES-like survey providing representative population-based objective clinical information. Some states and localities are moving in this direction. Currently four states receive funding from the DHDSP through the State Cardiovascular Health Examination Survey program to initiate state HANES-like surveys, but data are not yet available. NYC currently conducts a local version of the HANES that is a population-based, cross-sectional survey of noninstitutionalized NYC adult residents 20 years of age and older (Angell et al., 2008). The survey has allowed the NYC Department of Health and Mental Hygiene to monitor the health of NYC residents including the prevalence, awareness, treatment, and control of hypertension. SLHJs without the resources to implement a state-level HANES may need to identify other reliable population-based data sets, for example, health care quality reporting data, that could be used to monitor local hypertension trends.

6.4 The committee recommends that state and local public health jurisdictions assess their capacity to develop local HANES as a means to obtain local estimates of the prevalence, awareness, treatment, and control of hypertension. Further, if a program to reduce hypertension is a national goal, funding should be made available to assure that localities have relevant data that will assist them in addressing hypertension in their communities.

The committee recognizes that local financial constraints may not allow many SLHJs to move forward in this regard in the short term; thus, SLHJs may want to actively seek other reliable and available population-based data sets as a way to monitor local hypertension trends.

As a primary strategy, interventions in which public health dollars are used to directly deliver high-quality hypertension detection and treatment services are unlikely because of the cost of these interventions. Furthermore, direct interventions providing direct health care to individuals are most distant from the unique skills and value-added of state and local health agencies. But, because hypertension is treatable, SLHJs should consider how to use their limited resources to best leverage health care dollars for improved treatment and control of hypertension.

Public health agencies vary widely in their working relations and links with the health care providers in their jurisdictions. In some areas, linkages are strong and the SLHJ could play a valuable role in convening and advocating for improved treatment and care for persons with hypertension. But such activity will not be equally productive everywhere and will require a case-by-case assessment. Alternatively, SLHJs may be able to play an effective leadership and convening and brokering role in influencing community-wide health care practices, for example, through advocacy for incorporating measures of hypertension control in local or regional measures of health care quality. Assuring complementary lifestyle interventions (physical activity, weight management, healthy diet) in health care treatment protocols and linking these activities to community-based strategies through community health workers may be another important element of a local hypertension control program.

Systolic hypertension in the elderly is the most common form of uncontrolled hypertension in the United States. One area of special SLHJs activity relative to the hypertension health care delivery system may be to increase provider awareness of both prevalence and evidence of treatment effectiveness for moderate systolic hypertension in older patients and monitoring of provider performance in meeting Joint National Commission (JNC) treatment guidelines.

6.5 The committee recommends that state and local public health jurisdictions serve as conveners of health care system representatives, physician groups, purchasers of health care services, quality improvement organizations, and employers (and others) to develop a plan to engage and leverage skills and resources for improving the medical treatment of hypertension.

6.6 State and local public health jurisdictions should work with business coalitions and purchasing coalitions to remove economic barriers to effective antihypertensive medications for individuals who have difficulty accessing them.

6.7 State and local public health jurisdictions should promote and work with community health worker initiatives to ensure that prevention and control of hypertension is included in the array of services they provide and are appropriately linked to primary care services.

RESOURCES FOR HYPERTENSION PREVENTION AND CONTROL

The DHDSP has developed a comprehensive strategic plan that is not implementable in full with the current resources available. Considering the limited available resources, the committee has provided recommendations on priorities among the many possible activities laid out by the DHDSP. These recommendations have centered on population-based policy and system interventions in which funding can leverage other public health, health care, and private sector funding for improved prevention, treatment, and control of hypertension. The committee notes, in fact, there are fewer public health resources for hypertension prevention than for any other preventable risk factor underlying a disease burden of comparable magnitude. As an example, CDC funding for the Office on Smoking and Health is $106.2 million while funding for the Division for Heart Disease and Stroke Prevention is $54.1 million; this funding supports activities related to not only hypertension but also stroke and cardiovascular disease in general. Federal under funding of and insufficient attention to hypertension relative to the preventable burden of disease has played out at the state and local level as well. In general, states and localities have not invested in public health chronic disease prevention programs to the extent to which they have invested in communicable diseases (Frieden, 2004; Georgeson et al., 2005; Porterfield et al., 2009; Prentice and Flores, 2007). The evidence presented in Chapter 4 indicates there is potential for a substantial preventive, nonpharmacologic, non-health care, population-based policy and system strategy to be implemented at the federal, state, and local levels. There is also room for substantial improvement in health care diagnosis and treatment as discussed in Chapter 5. Implementation of the strategy, however, will be hampered by limited resources. With the nation's attention now focused on health care reform in general and specifically on the potential role of prevention, there is also the opportunity to advocate for increased financing for hypertension prevention and control.

In an era of declining resources and conflicting priorities for public health, taking on any new challenges needs careful consideration. But given the disease and economic burden associated with hypertension, and in this climate of health care reform and increasing attention to prevention, there is great public health opportunity and no better time to rise to the challenge.

6.8 The committee recommends that Congress give priority to assuring adequate resources for implementing a broad suite of population-based policy and system approaches at the federal, state, and local levels that have the greatest promise to prevent, treat, and control hypertension.

The committee notes that it was hampered in fully understanding how DHDSP funds were used for hypertension prevention and control activities at the state level insomuch as many of these activities were embedded in larger stroke or cardiovascular prevention and control activities. Reporting of program activity and funding data was not sufficiently detailed to ascertain the degree of funding that was specifically related to hypertension prevention, treatment, and control. A vital component of DHDSP prioritization of activities must be budget allocation. Rational decisions about where in a portfolio the next dollar should be spent can only be made with good information about where current dollars are being spent. A gap analysis comparing current resource use against priorities is critical to assure adequate resources are devoted to the highest-priority areas.

Attendant to current funding and potential future funding for hypertension prevention, treatment, and control, systems need to be in place to track and measure current and new programs activities at the federal, state, and local levels. Such a system would help ensure that resources are appropriately aligned and outcomes are achieved.

6.9 The committee recommends that the Division for Heart Disease and Stroke Prevention develop resource accountability systems to track and measure all current and new state programs for the prevention, treatment, and control of hypertension that would allow for resources to be assessed for alignment with the population-based policy and systems strategy and for measuring the outcomes achieved.

The committee acknowledges that the recommendations proffered, if adopted, would result in a significant programmatic change for the DHDSP. To effectively support the change and maintain a population-based focus, new expertise and guidance may be required beyond that which may be available through the DHDSP's partnership with the National Forum for Heart Disease and Stroke Prevention.

6.10 The committee recommends that the Division for Heart Disease and Stroke Prevention identify and work with experts grounded in population-based approaches to provide guidance and assistance in designing and executing hypertension prevention and control efforts that focus on population-based policy and system change. These experts

could augment an existing advisory body or be drawn from an existing body with this expertise.

ENSURING SYSTEM ACCOUNTABILITY

The committee considered the results that could be expected if the population-based policy and systems approach to prevent and control hypertension were implemented, including the potential effect on the overall prevalence of hypertension in the population and on racial and ethnic disparities. This section outlines the committee's consideration of those issues and identifies potential outcomes and indicators. The committee's consideration of potential indictors was informed by the division's draft document on *Policy and System Outcome Indicators for State Heart Disease and Stroke Prevention, Priority Area: High Blood Pressure Control* (DHDSP, 2008).

The committee believes that attention to the high-priority areas it has identified would lead to a reduction in the prevalence of hypertension, improve the quality of care provided to individuals with hypertension and in the long term, and ultimately, reduce mortality and morbidity due to heart disease and stroke. In the short term, one visible impact would be strong federal, state, and local public health agency leadership that gives priority to reducing the prevalence of hypertension through population-based approaches integrated throughout agency activities, particularly those that target hypertension risk factors by reducing obesity, promoting health diets, and increasing physical activity. Active engagement and efforts by federal, state, and local jurisdictions to reduce sodium consumption, an area not typically addressed by parts of the governmental public health system, would be another short-term visible impact. Improved estimates of hypertension prevalence, awareness, treatment, and control for the population as a whole and subgroups of the population at the national, state, and local levels would be important results of efforts to improve surveillance and monitoring of hypertension trends. Similarly, through improved data collection, public health officials would have better estimates to monitor their progress in reducing dietary sodium consumption and the sodium content in food.

Improved blood pressure control, especially systolic blood pressure among the elderly, would be the result of strategies designed to address the factors contributing to poor physician adherence to JNC treatment guidelines. The effect of removing economic barriers to effective antihypertensive medications and employing the use of community health workers to provide community-based support for individuals with hypertension would be improved access to medications and supportive hypertension care for vulnerable populations. Finally, essentially all of the proposed interventions have the potential to reduce health disparities if they are implemented with this goal in mind. However, this goal may not be in the forefront by all; thus, continued monitoring of health disparities will be necessary.

Table 6-1 summarizes the committee's recommendations for high-priority areas and related short-term and intermediate outcomes, and potential indicators to measure the progress made in advancing the committee's high-priority areas. Decreased mortality and morbidity from heart disease and stroke are understood as the ultimate long-term indicators; as such, they are not included in the table due to space consideration. The table is divided into broad sections (e.g., Population-Based Recommendations to the CDC's Division for Heart Disease and Stroke Prevention (DHDSP) and State and Local Jurisdictions (SLHJs), System Approaches Targeting Individuals with Hypertension Directed to the CDC and SLHJs, etc.) and includes subgroups of recommendations under those headings. Outcomes and indicators found in adjacent columns do not tract directly across but correspond to the subgroup of recommendations. Recommendations for resources and accountability (6.8-6.10) are not included in the table.

HYPERTENSION AS A SENTINEL FOR SUCCESS OF THE PUBLIC HEALTH SYSTEM IN REDUCING HEALTH DISPARITIES

Hypertension may provide an opportunity unique in public health chronic disease prevention for program evaluation through outcome measurement. In contrast to most chronic disease outcomes, measurement of hypertension has a combination of key ideal characteristics, including: (1) objectivity, (2) low cost, (3) ease and reproducibility, and (4) rapid response to intervention. In this context, it provides a single, reliable outcome measure that can be linked to intervention process measures to rapidly inform program interventions. It is also an early objective outcome measure of multiple public health and medical interventions to increase healthy eating and physical exercise.

Hypertension is prevalent, preventable, treatable, easily measured, and rapidly changeable. As such, it is a potential sentinel indicator for assessing and testing broader approaches to reduce health disparities. Hypertension is a condition strongly influenced by underlying individual and community risk factors related to healthy eating and active living—risk factors driven by race and class in most communities today. The prevalence of hypertension may provide a relatively quick and objective measure of programs directed at these risk factors as well as underlying social determinants of health. Hypertension, while treatable, requires ongoing access to primary care for maximum effectiveness. Thus, it is also a potentially very good marker for access to and continuity of health care in a community. The

TABLE 6-1 Priority Recommendations

Population-Based Recommendations to the Division for Heart Disease and Stroke Prevention (DHDSP) and State and Local Public Health Jurisdictions (SLHJs)

Recommendations to Enhance Population-Based Efforts and to Strengthen Efforts Among CDC Units and Partners

Priority Recommendation	Short-Term Outcomes (or process input or outputs)	Short-Term Indicator	Intermediate Outcomes	Intermediate Indicators
4.1 The DHDSP should integrate hypertension prevention and control in programmatic efforts to effect system, environmental, and policy changes through collaboration with other CDC units and their external partners. High-priority programmatic activities on which to collaborate include interventions for: -reducing overweight and obesity, -promoting the consumption of a healthy diet, -increasing potassium-rich fruits and vegetables in the diet, and -increasing physical activity.	Better targeting and integration of hypertension prevention in other CDC unit programming	Budget allocated to population-based policy and system approaches by the CDC	Reduction of hypertension risk factors in the population	Prevalence of overweight/obesity Proportion of individuals who consume a healthy diet
	New CDC budget and programs dedicated to policy and program system change strategies for hypertension	Budget and plans for hypertension program integration into other CDC prevention activities	Reduced incidence of hypertension	Proportion of children and adults who participate regularly in physical activities
4.2 Population-based interventions to improve physical activity and food environments (typically the focus of other CDC units) should include an evaluation of their feasibility and effectiveness, and their specific impact on hypertension prevalence and control.	Greater collaboration among CDC units on population-based interventions to prevent hypertension	Number of CDC activities that include a focus on hypertension prevention and control	Data on feasibility and effectiveness of a broad range of interventions that contribute to the prevention of hypertension	Reduction in adverse lifestyle behaviors

4.3 The DHDSP should leverage its ability to shape state activities, through its grant making and cooperative agreements, to encourage state activities to shift toward population-based prevention of hypertension.	Prevention of hypertension integrated in other unit strategies to: reduce overweight and obesity, promote healthy diet, increase consumption of fruits and vegetables, increase physical activity	Number of federal, state, and community policy and environmental strategies implemented to control high blood pressure	Reduced prevalence of hypertension	Percent reduction in disparities in high blood pressure risk factors between general and priority populations
6.1 SLHJs should give priority to population-based approaches over individual-based approaches to prevent and control hypertension.		Number of SLHJs that have added hypertension program elements and focus to nonhypertension programs		
6.2 SLHJs should integrate hypertension prevention and control in programmatic efforts to effect system, environmental, and policy changes that will support healthy eating, active living, and obesity prevention. Existing and new programmatic efforts should be assessed to ensure they are aligned with populations, most likely to be affected by hypertension such as older populations, which are often not the target of these programs.	Strong federal, state, and local public health agency leadership that gives priority to reducing the prevalence of hypertension through population-based approaches integrated throughout agency activities	Number of SLHJs with comprehensive programs for population hypertension control programs		

continued

TABLE 6-1 Continued

Recommendations to Strengthen Leadership in Reducing Sodium Intake and Increasing Potassium Intake

Priority Recommendation	Short-Term Outcomes (or process input or outputs)	Short-Term Indicator	Intermediate Outcomes	Intermediate Indicators
4.4 The DHDSP should take active leadership in convening other partners in federal, state, and local government and industry to advocate for and implement strategies to reduce sodium in the American diet to meet dietary guidelines, which are currently less than 2,300 mg/day (equivalent to 100 mmol/day) for the general population and 1,500 mg/day (equivalent to 70 mmol/day) for blacks, middle-aged and older adults, and individuals with hypertension.	Aggressive actions at the federal, state, and local levels to reduce sodium consumption and sodium content in the diet	Proportion of states and localities with a strategic plan to reduce sodium intake and sodium content in food	Reduction of salt consumption by the American population	Mean population urinary sodium excretion level
	Development and implementation of federal, state, land ocal programs to reduce sodium intake	Federal, state, and local budgets and plans for programs to reduce sodium intake	Reduction of salt content in food	Proportion of individuals who consume five or more fruits and vegetables per day
			Reduced prevalence of hypertension	

6.3 SLHJs should immediately begin to consider developing a portfolio of dietary sodium reduction strategies that make the most sense for early action in their jurisdictions.	Number of states implementing new or expanded programs to increase potassium rich fruit and vegetable consumption	Increase in potassium rich fruit and vegetable consumption	Mean population urinary potassium excretion level
4.5 DHDSP should specifically consider as a strategy advocating for the greater use of potassium/sodium chloride combinations as a means of simultaneously reducing sodium intake and increasing potassium intake.	Development and implementation of programs to increase potassium intake	Budget and plans for programs for increasing potassium consumption	Reduction of hypertension risk factors in the population	Mean and median blood pressure levels

continued

TABLE 6-1 Continued

Recommendations to Improve the Surveillance and Reporting of Hypertension and Risk Factors

Priority Recommendation	Short-Term Outcomes (or process input or outputs)	Short-Term Indicator	Intermediate Outcomes	Intermediate Indicators
2.1 The DHDSP should identify methods to better use (analyze and report) existing data on the monitoring and surveillance of hypertension over time and develop norms for data collection, analysis, and reporting of future surveillance of blood pressure levels and hypertension. In developing better data collection methods and analyses, the DHDSP should increase and improve analysis and reporting of understudied populations including: children, racial and ethnic minorities, the elderly, and socioeconomic groups.	Guidance on methods for analyzing and reporting existing data for monitoring and surveillance of hypertension and future data collection methods and analyses	Improved estimates of hypertension prevalence, awareness, treatment, and control for the population as a whole and subgroups of the population (children, racial and ethnic minorities, the elderly, and socioeconomic groups) at the national, state, and local levels	Improved capacity for assessing and monitoring progress in hypertension prevention and control	Improved program design and implementation as a result of better data
6.4 SLHJs should assess their capacity to develop local HANES as a means to obtain local estimates of the prevalence, awareness, treatment, and control of hypertension. Further, if a program to reduce hypertension is a national goal, funding should be made available to assure that localities have relevant data that will assist them in addressing hypertension in their communities.	Increased number of state and localities with a NHANES-like survey	Number of states and localities with data systems that provide estimates of the prevalence, awareness, treatment, and control of hypertension for their jurisdictions	Access to local data on hypertension trends	Number of states and localities that are implementing program changes based on local surveillance and reporting information

| 4.6 The DHDSP and other CDC units, should explore methods to develop and implement data-gathering strategies that will allow for more accurate assessment and tracking of specific foods that are important contributors to dietary sodium intake by the American people. | Improved systems for measuring or estimating sodium content in food are designed and implemented | Availability of data on specific foods that are important contributors to dietary sodium intake by the American people | Data on high-sodium-containing foods are tracked and used to develop strategies for reduction | Percent of high content sodium products that have reduced their sodium content |
| 4.7 The DHDSP and other CDC units should explore methods to develop and implement data-gathering strategies that will allow for more accurate assessment and the tracking of population-level dietary sodium and potassium intake including the monitoring of 24-hour urinary sodium and potassium excretion. | Improved systems for measuring or estimating dietary sodium and potassium intake are designed and implemented | Availability of mean population dietary sodium and potassium intake at the national, state, and local levels | Data on dietary sodium consumption are available and used to target dietary sodium reduction programs | Reduction in mean dietary sodium intake |

continued

TABLE 6-1 Continued

System Change Recommendations Directed at Individuals with Hypertension

Recommendations to Improve the Quality of Care Provided to Individuals with Hypertension

Priority Recommendation	Short-Term Outcomes (or process input or outputs)	Short-Term Indicator	Intermediate Outcomes	Intermediate Indicators
5.1 The DHDSP should give high priority to conducting research to better understand the reasons behind poor physician adherence to current JNC guidelines. Once these factors are better understood, strategies should be developed to increase the likelihood that primary providers will screen for and treat hypertension appropriately, especially in elderly patients.	Better understanding of reasons behind poor physician adherence to JNC guidelines Targeted strategies to improve provider awareness, understanding, acceptance, and adherence to JNC treatment guidelines	Proportion of providers who measure and classify blood pressure according to JNC guidelines Proportion of providers who follow JNC pharmacologic therapies for treatment of hypertension	Improved rates of diagnosed, treated, and controlled patients, especially systolic blood pressure control among the elderly	Proportion of individuals with hypertension who have achieved blood pressure control

5.2 The DHDSP should work with The Joint Commission and the health care quality community to improve provider performance on measures focused on assessing adherence to guidelines for screening for hypertension, the development of a hypertension disease management plan that is consistent with JNC guidelines, and achievement of blood pressure control.	Partnerships with health care quality community focused on improving provider performance on quality measure for hypertension	Proportion of patients who receive provider-initiated prescription and follow-up of therapeutic lifestyle modifications Proportion of patients with uncontrolled high blood pressure who have documented provider initiated change in pharmaceutical intervention	Improvements in state- or local-level provider performance in quality measures associated with blood pressure treatment and control	Proportion of older individuals with systolic hypertension who receive appropriate treatment
6.5 SLHJs should serve as conveners of health care system representatives, physician groups, purchasers of health care services, quality improvement organizations, and employers (and others) to develop a plan to engage and leverage skills and resources for improving the medical treatment of hypertension	Development of local-level partnerships between SLHJs and health care representatives, physician groups, purchasers of health care services, quality improvement organizations, and employers around hypertension prevention and control	Development of local collaborative plans to address hypertension prevention, control, and treatment		Improvement in state reported diagnosis, treatment, and control rates

continued

TABLE 6-1 Continued

Recommendations to Remove Economic Barriers to Effective Antihypertensive Medications

Priority Recommendation	Short-Term Outcomes (or process input or outputs)	Short-Term Indicator	Intermediate Outcomes	Intermediate Indicators
5.3 The DHDSP should encourage the Centers for Medicare & Medicaid Services to recommend the elimination or reduction of deductibles for antihypertensive medications among plans participating under Medicare Part D, and work with state Medicaid programs and encourage them to eliminate deductibles and copayments for antihypertensive medications. The DHDSP should work with the pharmaceutical industry and its trade organizations to standardize and simplify applications for patient assistance programs that provide reduced-cost or free antihypertensive medications for low-income, underinsured, or uninsured individuals.	Reduced cost for effective antihypertensive medication, especially among the poor, elderly, and those without health insurance coverage	Out-of-pocket costs for antihypertensive medications by insurance and economic status	Improved adherence to antihypertensive medications especially in the poor, elderly, and those without health insurance coverage Improved hypertension control, especially in the poor, elderly, and those without health insurance coverage	Prevalence of controlled hypertension, especially in the poor, elderly, and those without health insurance coverage Proportion of patients who adhere to antihypertensive medication regimens Degree of disparity in blood pressure control between general and priority populations

5.4 The DHDSP should collaborate with leaders in the business community to educate them about the impact of reduced patient costs on antihypertensive medication adherence and work with them to encourage employers to leverage their health care purchasing power to advocate for reduced deductibles and copayments for antihypertensive medications in their health insurance benefits packages.	Partnerships between the DHDSP and business community focused on reducing out-of-pocket costs for antihypertensive medications	Out-of-pocket costs for antihypertensive medications for worksite employees	Improved adherence to antihypertensive medications among employees	Proportion of employees who adhere to antihypertensive medication regimens Degree of disparity in blood pressure control between general and priority employee populations
6.6 SLHJs should work with business coalitions and purchasing coalitions to remove economic barriers to effective antihypertensive medications for individuals who have difficulty accessing them.	Partnerships between SLHJs and business community focused on reducing out-of-pocket costs for antihypertensive medications			

continued

TABLE 6-1 Continued

Recommendations to Provide Community Support for Individuals with Hypertension

Priority Recommendation	Short-Term Outcomes (or process input or outputs)	Short-Term Indicator	Intermediate Outcomes	Intermediate Indicators
5.5 The DHDSP should work with state partners to ensure that existing community health worker programs include a focus on the prevention and control of hypertension. In the absence of such programs, the DHDSP should work with state partners to develop programs of community health workers who would be deployed in high-risk communities to help support healthy living strategies that include a focus on hypertension.	Design and implementation of new or enhanced community health worker programs targeting hypertension control	Budget allocated to development or enhancement of community health worker programs	Improved hypertension control in communities served by community health worker programs	Prevalence of uncontrolled hypertension in communities served by community health workers
		Number of community health worker programs targeting hypertension		Degree of reduction in disparities in blood pressure control between general population and populations served by community health workers
6.7 SLHJs should promote and work with community health worker initiatives to ensure that prevention and control of hypertension is included in the array of services they provide and are appropriately linked to primary care services.				

combination of these two elements or drivers of hypertension potentially increases the likelihood that standard public health interventions may increase rather than decrease disparities, as has often been the case in tobacco reduction interventions. SLHJs should consider hypertension as a sentinel measure for evaluation of the effectiveness of a range of disparity-reducing activities, especially place-based strategies tackling conditions through community policy interventions.

Hypertension is also a disease of aging, becoming increasingly prevalent as individuals grow older. From the perspectives of the proportion affected, attention must be directed toward groups with the highest prevalence. But from the perspective of the individual, hypertension in younger age groups has a greater potential for causing premature morbidity and mortality, and therefore so special attention needs to be paid to this risk population.

REFERENCES

Angell, S. Y., R. K. Garg, R. C. Gwynn, L. Bash, L. E. Thorpe, and T. R. Frieden. 2008. Prevalence, awareness, treatment, and predictors of control of hypertension in New York City. *Circulation: Cardiovascular Quality and Outcomes* 1(1):46-53.

DHDSP (Division for Heart Disease and Stroke Prevention). 2008. *Policy and system outcome indicators for state heart disease and stroke prevention, priority area: High blood pressure control.* Atlanta, GA: Centers for Disease Control and Prevention.

Frieden, T. R. 2004. Asleep at the switch: Local public health and chronic disease. *American Journal of Public Health* 94(12):2059-2061.

Georgeson, M., L. Thorpe, M. Merlino, T. Frieden, J. Fielding, and The Big Cities Health Coalition. 2005. Shortchanged? An assessment of chronic disease programming in major US city health departments. *Journal of Urban Health* 82(2):183-190.

IOM (Institute of Medicine). 2002. *The future of the public's health in the 21st century.* Washington, DC: The National Academies Press.

———. 2007. *Progress in preventing childhood obesity: How do we measure up?* Washington, DC: The National Academies Press.

———. 2009. *Local government actions to prevent childhood obesity.* Washington, DC: The National Academies Press.

National Centre for Social Research. 2008. *An assessment of dietary sodium levels among adults (aged 19-64) in the UK general population in 2008, based on analysis of dietary sodium in 24 hour urine samples.* http://www.food.gov.uk/multimedia/pdfs/sodium report08.pdf (accessed January 15, 2010).

Porterfield, D. S., J. Reaves, T. R. Konrad, B. J. Weiner, J. M. Garrett, M. Davis, C. W. Dickson, M. Plescia, J. Alexander, and E. L. Baker, Jr. 2009. Assessing local health department performance in diabetes prevention and control—North Carolina, 2005. *Preventing Chronic Disease* 6(3):A87.

Prentice, B., and G. Flores. 2007. Local health departments and the challenge of chronic disease: Lessons from California. *Preventing Chronic Disease* 4(1):A15.

The City of New York. 2009. Statement of health organiztions and public agencies. http://www.nyc.gov/html//doh/html/cardio/cardio-salt-coalition.shtml (accessed December 18, 2009).

A

Committee Member Biographies

David W. Fleming, M.D. *(Chair, March 2009-February 2010)*, is the Director of the Department of Public Health in Seattle & King County. Previously in his career, Dr. Fleming directed the Bill & Melinda Gates Foundation's Global Health Strategies Program, served as the Deputy Director of the Centers for Disease Control and Prevention in Atlanta, Georgia, and was the State Epidemiologist for the Oregon Health Division. Dr. Fleming has published on a wide range of public health issues, and he has served on multiple boards and commissions, including the Board of the Global Alliance for Vaccines and Immunization. He has served on numerous Institute of Medicine (IOM) committees, including the Committee on Training Physicians for Public Health Careers, the Committee on the Elimination of Tuberculosis in the United States, and the Panel on Performance Measures for Data and Public Health Performance Partnership Grants. Dr. Fleming received his M.D. from the State University of New York Upstate Medical Center in Syracuse. He is board certified in internal medicine and preventive medicine and serves on the faculty of the Departments of Public Health at both the University of Washington and Oregon Health Sciences University.

Howard Koh, M.D., M.P.H. *(Chair, January-March 2009)*, was the Harvey V. Fineberg Professor of the Practice of Public Health and Associate Dean for Public Health Practice in the Department of Health Policy and Management at the Harvard School of Public Health while serving on this committee. Dr. Koh's research interests include exploring community-based strategies to reduce cancer disparities and promote cancer prevention and early detection, as well as tobacco control. Previously, he served as Massachusetts Commissioner of Public Health to advance projects with a broad array of state and national organizations including the Centers for Disease Control and Prevention and the National Cancer Institute. He is a member of the IOM and has participated in a number of IOM activities. Dr. Koh received his M.D. from Yale University and his M.P.H. from the Boston University School of Public Health.

Ana V. Diez-Roux, M.D., Ph.D., M.P.H., is Professor of Epidemiology, Director of the Center for Integrative Approaches to Health Disparities, and Associate Director of the Center for Social Epidemiology and Population Health at the University of Michigan's School of Public Health. Her research interests include social epidemiology, cardiovascular disease epidemiology, air pollution and cardiovascular risk, race and ethnic disparities, and systems approaches in population health. She has published extensively on a variety of public health issues, including the relationship between communities and cardiovascular risk factors and exposure to particulate matter and subsequent development of atherosclerosis, among others. Dr. Diez-Roux earned a Ph.D. and M.P.H. from the Johns Hopkins University School of Hygiene and Public Health. She also earned an M.D. from the University of Buenos Aires in 1985.

Jiang He, M.D., Ph.D., is Joseph S. Copes Chair and Professor in the Department of Epidemiology at Tulane University. His research interests include the etiology and prevention of cardiovascular disease, kidney disease, and stroke; ethnic and gender differences in chronic disease and international comparisons of disease; and gene and environment interaction on hypertension and other cardiovascular disease. He has published extensively on a variety of topics including cardiovascular disease risk factors. Dr. He earned his Ph.D. from the Johns Hopkins School of Public Health, his Dr.Med.Sc. from Peking Union Medical College, and his M.D. from Jiangxi Medical College in Jiangxi, China.

Kathy Hebert, M.D., M.P.H., M.M.M., is an Associate Professor of Medicine at the University of Miami, Miller School of Medicine. She received her medical degree from Louisiana State University School of Medicine and completed fellowships in cardiology/nuclear medicine from the Alton Ochsner Medical Foundation in Louisiana. Dr. Hebert also holds an M.M.M. degree from the Tulane School of Public Health and an M.P.H. degree from the Harvard School of Public Health. Before joining the University of Miami, Dr. Hebert was the state task force director for congestive heart failure disease management at the Louisiana State University Health

Care Services Division and Director of Cardiology at the Chabert Medical Center in Louisiana.

Corinne Husten, M.D., M.P.H., was the Vice President for Programs and Policy at the Partnership for Prevention while working on this committee. Partnership for Prevention is a nonprofit devoted to improving the lives of all Americans through prevention. Previously, she served as Chief of the Epidemiology Branch and as Acting Director of the Office on Smoking and Health at the Centers for Disease Control and Prevention (CDC). Some of her accomplishments include serving as the scientific lead for developing the Healthy People 2010 tobacco control objectives, leading the release of the Surgeon General's report on second-hand smoke, developing "Best Practices" for tobacco prevention and control, serving on the guideline panel for the Public Health Service "Treating tobacco use and dependence" guideline, providing technical assistance to the Community Preventive Services Task Force guideline recommendations on tobacco, and helping plan tobacco-free campus initiatives at the CDC and Department of Health and Human Services. Dr. Husten received her M.D. from Georgetown University School of Medicine and her M.P.H. from the Johns Hopkins University School of Hygiene and Public Health. She is currently Senior Medical Advisor for the Center for Tobacco Products at the Food and Drug Administration.

Sherman A. James, Ph.D., is the Susan B. King Professor of Public Policy Studies and also Professor of Sociology and Community and Family Medicine at Duke University. Dr. James, a social epidemiologist, studies the social determinants of racial disparities in health and health care, particularly in cardiovascular disease and diabetes. He is a member of the IOM (elected in 2000) and served on the Committee for Review and Assessment of the National Institutes of Health's (NIH's Strategic Plan to Reduce and Ultimately Eliminate Health Disparities. Dr. James earned his Ph.D. in social psychology from Washington University in St. Louis.

Thomas G. Pickering, M.D., D.Phil., was the Director of the Behavioral Cardiovascular Health and Hypertension Program at Columbia University Medical Center. Dr. Pickering's extensive research focuses on hypertension, psychosocial factors and cardiovascular disease, and delivery of effective care. His research contributions include the recognition of white coat hypertension as a clinically important entity of behavioral origin, the role of job strain in the development of hypertension, and the use of ambulatory and home blood pressure monitoring for evaluating the causes and consequences of hypertension. He has authored more than 550 scientific articles and chapters and recently served on the IOM Committee on Gulf War and Health: Physiologic, Psychologic, and Psychosocial Effects of Deployment-

Related Stress. Dr. Pickering served on numerous editorial boards of hypertension and behavioral medicine journals. In addition, he has served on several NIH task forces. He received his M.D. from Middlesex Hospital Medical School in London and his D.Phil. from Linacre College, Oxford University.

Geoffrey Rosenthal, M.D., Ph.D., is a pediatric cardiologist and currently a Professor of Pediatrics and Director of the Pediatric Heart Program at the Department of Pediatrics, Cardiology Division, University of Maryland Medical Center in Baltimore, MD. Dr. Rosenthal was previously the Director of the Pediatric Cardiovascular Research group at the Cleveland Clinic. Dr. Rosenthal has served on numerous committees including the Pediatric Advisory Committee for the Food and Drug Administration and as co-chair of the Quality Improvement Working Group of the Section on Adult Congenital and Pediatric Cardiology of the American College of Cardiology. He received his M.D. and Ph.D. in epidemiology from the University of Maryland School of Medicine.

Walter C. Willett, M.D., Dr.P.H., is the Fredrick John Stare Professor of Epidemiology and Nutrition in the Departments of Nutrition and Epidemiology at the Harvard School of Public Health. Dr. Willett is also the Chair of the Department of Nutrition. Dr. Willett's research primarily involves the investigation of dietary factors, using epidemiologic approaches, in the cause and prevention of cardiovascular disease, cancer, and other important conditions. Fundamental to this work has been the development of methods to measure dietary intake in large populations. In addition, Dr. Willett continues to work on the development and evaluation of biological markers of dietary intake, particularly using plasma and toenail samples. These biological indicators are primarily utilized in nested case control studies using the large specimen banks collected prospectively as part of ongoing studies. Dr. Willett is a member of the IOM. Dr. Willett received his M.D. from the University of Michigan in 1970 and his Dr.P.H. from the Harvard School of Public Health in 1980.

B

Agendas of Public Meetings Held by the Committee on Public Health Priorities to Reduce and Control Hypertension

FIRST PUBLIC MEETING

January 8, 2009
Room 109, Keck Building
Washington, DC

Welcome, Opening Remarks, and Introductions
Howard Koh, M.D.
Committee Chair

Historical Perspective of Hypertension Control
Aram Chobanian, M.D.
President Emeritus
Boston University

Charge to the Committee
Darwin Labarthe, M.D., M.P.H., Ph.D., FAHA
Director, Division for Heart Disease and Stroke Prevention
Centers for Disease Control and Prevention

Current Strategies for Hypertension Education and Control
Eduardo Ortiz, M.D., M.P.H.
Senior Medical Officer
Hypertension Guideline Program
National Heart, Lung, and Blood Institute (NHLBI)
National Institutes of Health

City Health Department Perspective
Sonia Angell, M.D., M.P.H.
Director
Cardiovascular Disease Prevention and Control Program
New York City Department of Health and Mental Hygiene

American Heart Association
Daniel Jones, M.D., FAHA
Director
Herbert G. Langfor Professor of Medicine
University of Mississippi School of Medicine
Mark Schoeberl
Executive Vice President – Advocacy
American Heart Association

Association of State and Territorial Health Officials
Susan Cooper, M.S.N., R.N.
Commissioner, Tennessee Department of Health
Chair, ASTHO's Prevention Policy Committee

Open Microphone and General Discussion

Adjourn Open Session

SECOND PUBLIC MEETING

April 9, 2009
Room 110, Keck Building
Washington, DC

Welcome, Opening Remarks, and Introductions
David Fleming, M.D.
Committee Chair

Lessons Learned from the National High Blood Pressure Education Program
Ed Roccella, Ph.D., M.P.H.
Retired Program Coordinator
National Heart, Lung, and Blood Institute
National Institutes of Health

Hypertension Detection and Follow-up Program and ALLHAT
Barry Davis, M.D., Ph.D.
Director of the Coordinating Center for Clinical Trials
University of Texas School of Public Health

CDC Hypertension Program and Budget
Kathryn Gallagher
Associate Director for Strategic Planning,
Partnerships and External Relations
Division of Heart Disease and Stroke Prevention
Centers for Disease Control and Prevention

Michael Schooley, M.P.H.
Chief, Applied Research and Evaluation Branch
Division of Heart Disease and Stroke Prevention
Centers for Disease Control and Prevention

Discussion of Data from CDC NHANES Analysis
Yuling Hong, M.D., Ph.D.
Associate Director for Science
Division of Heart Disease and Stroke Prevention
Centers for Disease Control and Prevention

Open Microphone and General Discussion

Adjourn Open Session

THIRD PUBLIC MEETING

June 1, 2009
Room 201, Keck Building
Washington, DC

Welcome, Opening Remarks, and Introductions
David Fleming, M.D.
Committee Chair

Racial and Ethnic Disparities in Hypertension
Richard Cooper, M.D.
Professor and Chair, Preventive Medicine and Epidemiology
Loyola University, Stritcher School of Medicine

Lessons Learned from the Minnesota Heart Health Program
Russell V. Luepker, M.D., M.S.
Mayo Professor
University of Minnesota, Epidemiology and Community Health

Effectiveness and Costs of Interventions to Lower Systolic Blood Pressure
Stephen Lim, Ph.D.
Assistant Professor of Global Health
Institute for Health Metrics and Evaluation, University of
Washington

Open Microphone and General Discussion

Adjourn Open Session

FIRST OPEN CONFERENCE CALL

March 9, 2009

Welcome
Howard Koh, M.D.
Committee Chair

Birth Cohort Evidence of Population Influences on Blood Pressure
David Goff, M.D., Ph.D.
Department of Epidemiology & Prevention
Division of Public Health Sciences
Wake Forest University

DASH Diet and OMNI Heart Trial
Frank Sacks, M.D.
Professor of Cardiovascular Disease Prevention
Department of Nutrition
Harvard School of Public Health

SECOND OPEN CONFERENCE CALL

March 30, 2009

Welcome
David Fleming, M.D.
Committee Chair

Centers for Disease Control and Prevention Presentation
    Darwin Labarthe, M.D., M.P.H., Ph.D., FAHA
    Director
    Division for Heart Disease and Stroke Prevention
    Centers for Disease Control and Prevention

State Health Programs
    Fred Petillo
    Heart Disease & Stroke Prevention Program
    Wisconsin Department of Health Service

C

A Public Health Action Plan to Prevent Heart Disease and Stroke

RECOMMENDATIONS

To help the public health community implement the Action Plan, specific recommendations were developed by five Expert Panels. These panels addressed the five essential components of the plan—taking action, strengthening capacity, evaluating impact, advancing policy, and engaging in regional and global partnerships. Their work was synthesized by a Working Group into 22 recommendations, which are presented here according to the Expert Panel that produced them.

Taking Action: Putting Present Knowledge to Work

1. Initiate policy development in CVH promotion and CVD prevention at national, state, and local levels to assure effective public health action against heart disease and stroke. In addition, evaluate policies in non-health sectors (e.g., education, agriculture, transportation, community planning) for their potential impact on health, especially with respect to CVD.

2. Act now to implement the most promising public health programs and practices for achieving the four goals for preventing heart disease and stroke, as distinguished by the Healthy People 2010 Heart and Stroke Partnership based on the different intervention approaches that apply. These goals are prevention of risk factors, detection and treatment of risk factors, early identification and treatment of heart attacks and strokes, and prevention of recurrent

cardiovascular events. Public health agencies and their partners must provide continuous leadership to identify and recommend new and effective interventions that are based on advances in program evaluation and prevention research and a growing inventory of "best practices."

3. Address all opportunities for prevention to achieve the full potential of preventive strategies. Such opportunities include major settings (schools, work sites, health care settings, communities, and families), all age groups (from conception through the life span), and whole populations, particularly priority populations (based on race/ethnicity, sex, disability, economic condition, or place of residence).

4. Emphasize promotion of desirable social and environmental conditions and favorable behavioral patterns in order to prevent the major CVD risk factors and assure the fullest attainable accessibility and use of quality health services for people with risk factors or who develop subclinical or overt CVD. These actions are integral to a comprehensive public health strategy for CVH promotion and CVD prevention.

Strengthening Capacity: Transforming the Organization and Structure of Public Health Agencies and Partnerships

5. Maintain or establish definable entities with responsibility and accountability for CVH programs within federal, state, and local public health agencies, including laboratory components.

6. Create a training system to develop and maintain appropriately trained public health workforces at national, state, and local levels. These workforces should have all necessary competencies to bring about policy change and implement programs to improve CVH promotion and decrease the CVD burden, including laboratory requirements.

7. Develop and disseminate model performance standards and core competencies in CVD prevention and CVH promotion for national, state, and local public health agencies, including their laboratories.

8. Provide ongoing access to technical assistance and consultation to state and local health agencies and partners for CVD prevention.

Evaluating Impact: Monitoring the Burden, Measuring Progress, and Communicating Urgency

9. Expand and standardize population-wide evaluation and surveillance data sources and activities to assure adequate assessment of CVD indicators and change in the nation's CVD burden. Examples include mortality, incidence, prevalence, disability, selected biomarkers, risk factors and risk behaviors, economic burden, community and environmental characteristics, current policies and programs, and sociodemographic factors (e.g., age, race/ethnicity, sex, and ZIP code).

10. Establish a network of data systems for evaluation of policy and program interventions that can track the progress of evolving best practices and signal the need for changes in policies and programs over time. This network would support the full development, collection, and analysis of the data needed to examine program effectiveness.

11. Develop the public health infrastructure, build personnel competencies, and enhance communication systems so that federal, state, and local public health agencies can communicate surveillance and evaluation results in a timely and effective manner.

Advancing Policy: Defining the Issues and Finding the Needed Solutions

12. Conduct and facilitate research by means of collaboration among interested parties to identify new policy, environmental, and sociocultural priorities for CVH promotion. Once the priorities are identified, determine the best methods for translating, disseminating, and sustaining them. Fund research to identify barriers and effective interventions in order to translate science into practice and thereby improve access to and use of quality health care and improve outcomes for patients with or at risk for CVD. Conduct economics research, including cost-effectiveness studies and comprehensive economic models that assess the return on investment for CVH promotion as well as primary and secondary CVD prevention.

13. Design, plan, implement, and evaluate a comprehensive intervention for children and youth in school, family, and community settings. This intervention must address dietary imbalances, physical inactivity, tobacco use, and other determinants in order to prevent development of risk factors and progression of atherosclerosis and high blood pressure.

14. Conduct and facilitate research on improvements in surveillance methods and data collection and management methods for policy development, environmental change, performance monitoring, identification of key indicators, and capacity development. Address population subgroups in various settings (schools, work sites, health care, and communities) at local, state, and national levels. Additionally, assess the impact of new technologies and regulations on surveillance systems and the potential benefit of alternative methods.

15. Conduct and support research to determine the most effective marketing messages and educational campaigns to create demand for heart-healthy options, change behavior, and prevent heart disease and stroke for specific target groups and settings. Create and evaluate economically viable CVD prevention ventures (e.g., in food production, manufacturing, marketing).

16. Initiate and strengthen training grants and other approaches, such as training workshops and supervised research opportunities, to build the competencies needed to implement the CVD prevention research agenda.

Engaging in Regional and Global Partnerships: Multiplying Resources and Capitalizing on Shared Experience

17. Engage with regional and global partners to mobilize resources in CVH promotion and CVD prevention, develop and implement global CVH policies, and establish or strengthen liaison with the partners identified in these recommendations.

18. Address inequalities in CVH among developed and developing countries, rich and poor people within countries, and men and women of all ages. Work with national and global partners to assess the impact of globalization and trade policies on global CVH.

19. Develop a strategy to promote use of the media to support.

20. Strengthen global capacity to develop, implement, and evaluate policy and program interventions to prevent and control heart disease and stroke. Involve all relevant parties—governmental and nongovernmental, public and private, and traditional and nontraditional partners—in a systematic and strategic approach.

21. Strengthen the global focus of public health agencies in the United States and their partners on CVH and increase their participation in partnerships intended to a) develop and implement standards for adequate monitoring of health, social, and economic indicators

and b) develop the ability to effectively disseminate and translate information into policy and action.

22. Promote and support research on implementing and evaluating CVH policy interventions in diverse settings where different social and economic development and health transition experiences offer contrasting conditions for testing new intervention approaches.

D

DHDSP Strategic Plan

Division for Heart Disease and Stroke Prevention
2007 Program Review

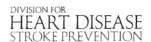

DIVISION FOR
HEART DISEASE
STROKE PREVENTION

Strategic Plan

Our Vision

A heart-healthy and stroke-free world

Our Mission

To serve as the nation's public health leader for achieving cardiovascular health for all and for eliminating the disparities in the burden of heart disease and stroke

Our Values

- ❖ Accountability
- ❖ Collaboration
- ❖ Communication
- ❖ Integrity
- ❖ Leadership
- ❖ Respect
- ❖ Service

Our Strategic Imperative

Lead the nation's public health efforts in achieving Healthy People 2010 heart disease and stroke goals:

1. Prevent risk factors for heart disease and stroke.
2. Increase detection and treatment of risk factors for heart disease and stroke.
3. Increase early identification and treatment of heart disease and stroke.
4. Prevent recurrences of heart attacks and strokes.

Division for Heart Disease and Stroke Prevention
2007 Program Review

Our Core Functions

Within each of our core functions, we are committed to being good stewards of public funds. We use the best science and resources available to develop interventions and programs that prevent, detect, and treat heart disease and stroke regardless of gender, disability, race, ethnicity, age, or socioeconomic status.

Evaluation

We evaluate programs, policies, and interventions regularly to ensure they are working as planned and producing the intended results. We support state program evaluation activities through evaluation research, technical assistance, resource development, and capacity building in evaluation.

Partnerships

We view partnerships with government agencies, states, academic researchers, public and private organizations, and other stakeholders essential to our work. Partnerships allow us to maximize our collective resources and bring about social environmental and policy changes that promote heart-healthy and stroke-free communities.

Programs

We provide funding, technical support, and resource materials to state health departments, tribes, and other partners to increase their program capacity. We develop and promote evidence-based strategies and interventions to help states and partners reduce health disparities and prevent heart disease and stroke throughout the lifespan.

Research

We engage in applied research to support evidence-based practice. Through our research, science translation, and resource development we help state and national health agencies implement public health strategies to address the burden of heart disease and stroke. Our technical support and extramural research funding extends CDC's capacity to improve cardiovascular health for all.

Resource Management

We work to ensure that our recruitment, retention, and training policies sustain a highly-skilled and diverse workforce. We promote integrity and accountability in all of our administrative transactions. We maintain an organizational structure that keeps abreast of current policies and procedures and helps us use our resources efficiently and effectively.

Surveillance

We track trends in cardiovascular risk factors and diseases and document differences in their distribution by age, gender, race/ethnicity, socioeconomic status, and geographic location. We analyze data patterns to identify groups of people most at risk of cardiovascular disease. We share our findings with colleagues, partners, and key stakeholders and promote collaboration in applying public health strategies to improve cardiovascular health.

Division for Heart Disease and Stroke Prevention
2007 Program Review

Our Goals and Strategies

GOAL 1: PREVENT RISK FACTORS FOR HEART DISEASE AND STROKE
Strategies:

1. Increase public awareness of the preventability of heart disease and stroke risk factors.

2. Enhance collaboration within the CDC, with federal/state/local agencies and with non-governmental organizations to mobilize prevention efforts.

3. Identify, evaluate, and disseminate strategies to prevent risk factors for heart disease and stroke, including adherence to guidelines.

4. Promote surveillance activities to measure the incidence of heart disease and stroke risk factors across the life stages.

5. Identify and address at-risk populations to prevent disparities associated with heart disease and stroke risk factors.

6. Improve and encourage policies and systems that promote heart-healthy behaviors and environments.

GOAL 2: INCREASE DETECTION AND TREATMENT OF RISK FACTORS FOR HEART DISEASE AND STROKE

Strategies:

1. Increase availability of preventive services, specifically lifestyle interventions, screenings, and appropriate medicines.

2. Identify populations experiencing disproportionately high rates of risk factors for heart disease and stroke and implement public health strategies to eliminate these disparities.

3. Identify, evaluate and disseminate strategies for implementation and adherence to guidelines for detection and treatment of heart disease and stroke risk factors.

Division for Heart Disease and Stroke Prevention
2007 Program Review

GOAL 3: INCREASE EARLY IDENTIFICATION AND TREATMENT OF HEART DISEASE AND STROKE

Strategies:

1. Increase capacity to monitor and address disparities and outcomes.

2. Improve quality of care for people who have suffered a heart attack or stroke:

   a) Promote public health policies that foster coordinated systems of care from recognition of symptoms through successful rehabilitation.
   b) Identify, evaluate, and disseminate strategies for early identification and treatment of heart attacks and strokes (e.g. awareness, timely action, transport, quality of acute care).
   c) Increase timely delivery of affordable, comprehensive treatment of heart attacks and strokes, especially among those experiencing disparities.

3. Increase public awareness of the signs and symptoms of heart attacks and strokes.

GOAL 4: DECREASE RECURRENCES OF CARDIOVASCULAR EVENTS.

Strategies:

1. Increase capacity to monitor, track and address disparities among people living with cardiovascular disease, including quality of life issues, adherence to guidelines, costs, economic indicators, functional status, and risk of developing mental incapacity.

2. Accelerate the translation of evidence-based science and guidelines.

3. Overcome barriers to preventing recurring events and long-term care by working with health care professionals and community organizations to reach people where they live, work, and play.

4. Increase availability of services to prevent recurring cardiovascular events, focusing on the public health perspective.

Division for Heart Disease and Stroke Prevention
2007 Program Review

GOAL 5: FOSTER A SKILLED AND ENGAGED PUBLIC HEALTH WORKFORCE TO ADDRESS
HEART DISEASE AND STROKE.

Strategies:

1. Increase skills and capacity of the public health workforce to prevent heart
   disease and stroke:

   a. Promote multiple methods to enhance skills and staff capacity.
   b. Promote a diverse workforce at all levels, including leadership.
   c. Promote recognition of excellence in the public health workforce to
      prevent heart disease and stroke.
   d. Promote collaboration across the public health workforce to prevent
      heart disease and stroke.

2. Create and maintain a positive Division work environment that promotes
   the following attributes:

   a. Respects and values cultural, educational, and professional diversity.
   b. Promotes a variety of learning opportunities to support professional staff
      development and skill building.
   c. Celebrates success.
   d. Provides a healthy physical environment.
   e. Provides effective systems, procedures, and communications to enhance
      work performance.
   f. Provides responsive management.

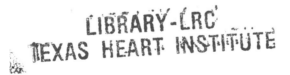